CANCER VIRUS

CANCER VIRUS

THE STORY OF EPSTEIN-BARR VIRUS

DOROTHY H. CRAWFORD,
ALAN RICKINSON,
& INGÓLFUR JOHANNESSEN

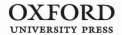

OXFORD
UNIVERSITY PRESS

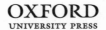

OXFORD
UNIVERSITY PRESS

Great Clarendon Street, Oxford, OX2 6DP,
United Kingdom

Oxford University Press is a department of the University of Oxford.
It furthers the University's objective of excellence in research, scholarship,
and education by publishing worldwide. Oxford is a registered trade mark of
Oxford University Press in the UK and in certain other countries

Published in the United States of America by Oxford University Press
198 Madison Avenue, New York, NY 10016, United States of America

British Library Cataloguing in Publication Data
Data available
Library of Congress Control Number: 2013948406
ISBN 978–0–19–965311–9
Printed in Italy by L.E.G.O. S.p.A.

CONTENTS

ACKNOWLEDGEMENTS

Cancer Virus records 50 years of scientific research on EBV since its discovery in 1964. Many thousands of scientists have played their part in this journey of discovery—too many to name here but we thank them all. We are particularly indebted to those who contributed interesting stories and quotes for the book, and to the following who gave their time to reminisce about their work on EBV: Arthur Ammann, George Ball, Guy de Thé, Volker Diehl, Anthony Epstein, Paul Farrell, Jim Jones, Hideaki Kikuta, Eva Klein, George Klein, Ian Magrath, Denis Moss, Dennis Wright, Zeng Yi, John Ziegler, and Harald zur Hausen.

We thank Denis Burkitt's wife, Olive, and their daughters for comments on the manuscript. We are also grateful to Latha Menon, our editor at Oxford University Press, and to William Alexander, Martin Allday, Jeanne Bell, Richard Boyd, Hunter Gray, Mark Pearson, Barbara Rickinson, Lesley Rowe, Martin Rowe, Alero Thomas, and Richard Vaughan for reading and providing helpful comments and suggestions on the manuscript.

PREFACE

With the fiftieth anniversary of the discovery of the first human tumour virus looming, we realized that the story of the discovery of Epstein-Barr virus (EBV) and the contents of Pandora's box that this revealed have never been related to a general audience. Aimed at the interested lay person, *Cancer Virus* takes the reader on a journey from the first key observation of a unique type of tumour in a Ugandan hospital in the 1950s to the landmark discovery of a virus in this tumour in a research laboratory in London in the 1960s. We then travel on to the US, Europe, Australia, China, and Japan, making more discoveries relating to this virus. Along the way we meet the key players involved, starting with Denis Burkitt, the Irish surgeon who was working in Uganda when he noticed a previously unrecognized but extremely common childhood tumour now called Burkitt Lymphoma. It was from the cells of this tumour that Anthony Epstein, a research virologist, and Yvonne Barr, a research assistant at the Middlesex Hospital in London, isolated the cancer virus of our title that now bears their names.

Since then the quest to prove that EBV is indeed a cancer virus, and to understand how those cancers arise, has involved many fascinating characters and several twists of fate. En route, even more EBV-related diseases, including several different types of cancer, have come to light. The discovery of EBV and the work that it inspired opened the door to a new science—the link between viruses and human tumours. Today this is a hugely important area of medical research involving thousands of clinicians and scientists across the fields of cell and molecular biology, genetics, epidemiology, immunology, and vaccine design.

All three authors of *Cancer Virus* are, or have been, EBV researchers who have watched its history unfold. The story in the book is our interpretation of the key events in that history. Inevitably many essential findings, the building blocks that set the stage for these events and the individual researchers who made those findings, have been glossed over in the interests of brevity; we apologize if this causes offence. In the division of labour, Dorothy Crawford and Alan Rickinson wrote the text while Ingólfur Johannessen carried out extensive interviews with key EBV researchers.

As far as possible we have avoided using technical terms but inevitably some have crept in that were essential for a clear understanding of the research that generated certain important discoveries. These terms are explained in the text, and there is also a glossary of terms at the end of the book that contains more detailed information. There is a simple timeline of key discoveries at the end of the book.

LIST OF FIGURES

Introduction

L ondon in the early 1960s: change was in the air. As the decade
unfolded, the young embraced a future seemingly full of possibilities. Artists, musicians, and designers flocked to the city and 'The
Swinging Sixties' was born.

Less trumpeted, yet just as important, a scientific revolution was
also under way, with London as an exciting and innovative international centre for medical research. Among the many scientific
breakthroughs of the time, there was one that epitomizes the spirit
of the age. An idea that was original, iconoclastic, and *so* contrary
to conventional wisdom that it had to fight for acceptance all the
way. Yet it had a kernel of truth that, 50 years later, has come to full
fruition.

The idea was that certain types of human cancer, one of the most
feared diseases, might be caused by a virus infection. Everyone was
familiar with viruses causing acute diseases like influenza or measles
from which most people soon recover. But it seemed fanciful that a
virus, just a tiny, inert particle, described by Sir Peter Medawar as 'a
piece of bad news wrapped up in protein',[1] could also cause a chronic,
progressive, life-threatening illness like cancer—a disease that everyone knew was not infectious.

That kind of conventional wisdom did not deter Anthony Epstein,
a medical researcher working at the Middlesex Hospital Medical

School. He was fascinated by earlier reports of 'infectious agents' causing cancer in certain laboratory animals, reports that many dismissed as rare curiosities with no general relevance to humans. But if under special circumstances viruses could cause cancer in animals, then why *not* in humans?

Epstein had trained at the Rockefeller Institute in New York, where scientists were beginning to look at cells with the electron microscope. With this instrument, much more powerful than a conventional light microscope, researchers could see a whole new world of sub-cellular structures, including viruses. Epstein reasoned that if some human cancers were caused by viruses he might be able to see them in the cancer cells using an electron microscope.

That was all well and good, but where to start? There are many types of cancer, probably all caused by different combinations of factors, so how to find one that might, just might, involve a virus?

At this point one of those coincidences occurred that lie at the heart of so many scientific breakthroughs. A doctor from Mulago Hospital in Uganda, Denis Burkitt, was visiting London in 1961, lecturing about a childhood cancer, later to become known as Burkitt Lymphoma. He had first seen a child with this tumour during his daily work in Uganda, but at the time it was unknown in the West. Burkitt then went on to show that this cancer was common in children throughout sub-Saharan Africa, but only in areas with high rainfall and high temperature. When Epstein heard Burkitt's lecture at the Middlesex Hospital he immediately thought 'A cancer which is restricted by temperature and rainfall: that's where to look for a cancer virus!'

From that chance encounter came the discovery, by Epstein and his research assistant, Yvonne Barr, of the virus that is now called the Epstein-Barr virus (EBV). They did indeed find the virus in Burkitt Lymphoma cells by electron microscopy—the first human virus ever to be discovered by that technique, and the first human cancer virus.

Today we know that EBV is not just linked to Burkitt Lymphoma but plays an important part in the development of at least five other types of human cancer. Many of these occur worldwide but, like Burkitt Lymphoma, with varying frequencies in different human populations. Interestingly, as well as being a cancer virus, EBV also causes the infectious disease, infectious mononucleosis (or glandular fever), which is common in the affluent Western world yet rare elsewhere. The same virus is now increasingly being linked to another disease with a similar preponderance for affluent societies, namely multiple sclerosis.

Who would have thought that a virus first seen under the electron microscope in a cancer from an African child would have such worldwide significance? *Cancer Virus* traces the story of EBV from those early days in sixties London to the present time, a journey full of surprises, setbacks, and personal drama, and a real insight into how circumstances and chance can shape the world of scientific discovery.

1

Out of Africa

The trail that led to the discovery of the first human tumour virus began in 1957 when Denis Burkitt, an Irish surgeon working in Uganda, identified the tumour that now bears his name—Burkitt Lymphoma. His meticulous descriptions of the tumour's remarkable clinical aspects and his tenacious pursuit of its geographical distribution made for a fascinating story that caught the attention of the researchers who eventually found the virus. This discovery heralded a profound change in thinking about the causes of cancer worldwide. Since 1964 several other human cancer-associated viruses have been identified, so that we now know that viruses are involved in the causation of around 10 per cent of all cases of human cancer.

At the height of his fame in the 1970s and 1980s, Burkitt (Figure 1) was feted the world over. Showered with prestigious prizes and medals, awarded numerous honorary degrees and fellowships, he was in constant demand to give lectures—always delivered with humour, panache and the timing of a natural actor. Yet Burkitt came from a very different background; a small town in rural Ireland. He was born in Enniskillen, County Fermanagh, Ireland, in 1911, the elder son of James Burkitt, from Donegal, and Gwendoline Hill from County Cork. James Burkitt was the County Surveyor for Fermanagh, but obviously had a natural interest in biology, and in the end was better known for his hobby—bird watching. He was the first to ring birds so that each

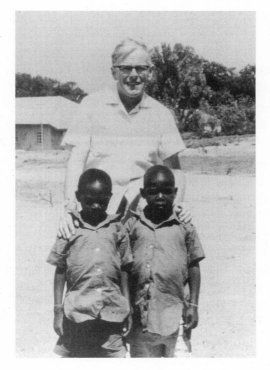

FIGURE 1 Denis Burkitt with two young patients

could be identified and studied in detail. He spent years observing the
goings-on of individual robins in his 10-acre garden: mapping their
territories, tracking their movements, and spotting their nest sites. In a
lifetime of close scrutiny he discovered that each robin has its own ter-
ritory that is so jealously guarded that fights against imposters are not
unusual, sometimes even ending in death for one of the combatants.
Burkitt senior was the first to show that these colourful and suppos-
edly friendly little birds are in fact the bullies of the garden's avian
community, and in doing so he became a legend in the world of orni-
thology.[2] It was this same attention to detail that led his son Denis to
make his own ground-breaking discoveries.

Within the family home two strong influences clearly laid the foundations for the young Burkitt's future life. The first of these was service to the British Empire where Burkitt had three paternal uncles living and working: one was a surgeon in East Africa, while the other two were in India, where one became Governor of Madras, the other Chief Engineer to the Punjab. While on leave back home these uncles must have regaled the family with stories from far-flung lands that inspired Burkitt as he grew up. On one occasion the surgeon uncle removed Denis' and his brother Robin's tonsils and adenoids on the kitchen table—clearly not an event that put them off medicine as both boys later became doctors.

The second enduring influence was that of religion. Both Burkitt's parents had a strong Christian faith and this influence obviously took root in the young Burkitt. To quote from his obituary: 'An unshakable belief in divine guidance and the efficacy of prayer lasted from these early days throughout Denis Burkitt's life and resulted in daily bible reading, the display of biblical texts in each of his successive offices, and abstinence from alcohol.'[3]

In 1929, Burkitt entered Trinity College Dublin to study engineering. But during his first year he believed that he had received a divine calling to become a doctor and so switched to studying medicine. After qualifying in 1935 he went to England to train and practise as a surgeon. Soon after war broke out in 1939 Burkitt was similarly moved to join the British army. So in 1940 he applied to join the Royal Army Medical Corp, but at that time they did not need surgeons and so his application was rejected. However, in early 1941 Burkitt again applied but was again rejected, this time because an accident at school at the age of 11 had left him with only one eye—a handicap that he overcame so effectively that few even suspected it. He was eventually accepted by the Medical Corp in May 1941 and spent the next two years training at army hospitals in the south of England.

Then in 1943 Burkitt was posted to East Africa where he served with African troops in Kenya and Somaliland. While on leave he visited friends in Uganda and here he decided that his life's vocation was 'in helping the people of Uganda both medically and spiritually'.[4] So it was that after demobilization in 1946 Burkitt joined the Colonial Service and six months later he was on his way to Lira Hospital in Lango District, Uganda, leaving his wife, Olive, at home in England, pregnant with their first child.

Burkitt boarded a ship bound for the port of Mombasa in Kenya, and then took the train to Kampala, capital of Uganda. From there he travelled by pickup truck to Lira, a journey of some 220 miles. Six months later Olive undertook this arduous journey with their baby daughter. When she arrived at Lira she had to adapt to the primitive living conditions—no piped water, a bucket served as a toilet, and light was provided by hurricane lamps. But she apparently made the best of it and soon made friends. Even in this remote place the British had all the usual traditional expatriate entertainments—golf, tennis, coffee mornings, and evenings at 'the club'.[5]

Burkitt, describing himself as a 'simple bush surgeon', ran a 100-bedded bush hospital in Lira assisted by just one African doctor. The workload was enormous: in the first year alone he increased the number of surgical operations from 17 to over 600. He and his family were happy in Lira, but had been there for less than two years when, in 1948, he received a telegram informing him that he had been posted to Mulago Hospital, the Makerere University College teaching hospital in Kampala. At the time, this hospital was expanding rapidly and the workload was even heavier than at Lira. Burkitt headed one of three surgical units and during his first 10 years at Mulago Hospital he made many improvements to the surgical services. However, it was in 1957 that a chance observation changed the direction of his career from 'simple bush surgeon' to medical superstar.

This transformation began when Hugh Trowell, an eminent physician and head of medical services at Mulago Hospital, asked Burkitt, as the duty surgeon at the time, to look at a patient who was puzzling him. This was a 5-year-old boy with swellings of his jaws. Many years later Burkitt recalled: 'His face was massively swollen, with bizarre lesions involving both sides of his upper and lower jaws. I had never seen anything like it. The teeth were loose and the features grossly distorted.'[6] Burkitt knew that single jaw tumours were common in Ugandan children (Figure 2), and thought to be some kind of sarcoma—that is a tumour of soft tissue such as muscle or nerve. Indeed he had operated on several of these jaw tumours, although he had never followed them up to find out how they fared. But he could shed no light on the diagnosis in this case because of the involvement of all four quadrants of the jaw. Thinking that it must either be an infection or a very unusual tumour, he took a biopsy, but unfortunately this too proved inconclusive. So, having made detailed notes on the case and taken photographs of the child's swollen face, Burkitt considered it to be 'another of the curiosities one had to become accustomed to seeing from time to time in Africa'.[7]

And this is where the story might have rested had Burkitt not visited the district hospital at Jinja on the shores of Lake Victoria a few weeks later. Here, while doing a ward round, he happened to glance

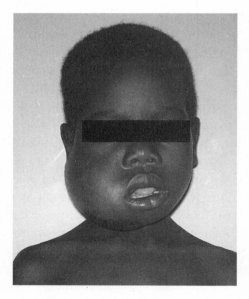

FIGURE 2 A typical case of Burkitt Lymphoma

out of the window and saw a small boy with a similar grossly swollen face sitting on the grass beside his mother. 'My interest was rivetted immediately. A curiosity can occur once, but two cases indicate more than a curiosity.'[8]

Now Burkitt's attention was truly aroused. Perhaps like his father with the robins, he would not rest until he had got to the bottom of the puzzle. He examined the second child thoroughly and found that, in addition to the jaw lesions, he had a lump in his abdomen. Burkitt immediately asked himself—could this be linked to the jaw swellings? To find the answer Burkitt pored over old hospital case notes and autopsy reports. Surprisingly, this revealed that the jaw swellings were frequently associated with tumours in a wide variety of organs, commonly the kidneys, ovaries, adrenal glands, and less often, the liver. Other tumour sites included the eyes, orbits, testes, thyroid gland, and long bones. On occasions the spinal cord was involved, causing paraplegia. The link between all these tumours had previously been missed because, while the jaw tumours were labelled sarcomas, the others were diagnosed as tumours common to the organs in which they arose. For example those in the eye were labelled retinoblastomas, those in the bones osteosarcomas and so on.

Burkitt's first breakthrough was the hunch that these disparate tumours were all part of the same disease. With this realization, he wrote his first scientific paper on the subject, describing 38 patients seen at Mulago and surrounding district hospitals. The report entitled *A sarcoma involving the jaws in African children* was published in the *British Journal of Surgery* in 1958.[9] In the publication he described cases with single or multiple tumours in the jaw and co-existing abdominal tumours, and discussed their bizarre presenting symptoms. With regard to the multiple jaw tumours, he thought it unlikely that one of the masses represented the primary tumour that had subsequently spread to the other affected sites because no known mode of spread existed between the four quadrants of the jaw. Equally, spread from a primary tumour in the jaw or abdomen to multiple abdominal organs was very unusual. In fact most other tumours first spread to local lymph glands, but with this tumour these glands were very rarely involved. So the question of how this clinical presentation came about left Burkitt mystified.

Burkitt's report attracted very little attention at the time, probably because it was published in a specialist journal read mainly by surgeons. However, several years later it became a citation classic. His discovery generated a host of new questions in Burkitt's mind: what was the nature of the disease and where was the primary tumour? How common was it? Was it a new disease or just newly recognized? With the help of colleagues, Burkitt wasted no time in finding answers to these questions.

First, Gregory O'Conor and Jack Davies, both pathologists at Mulago Hospital, re-examined tumours from all the different sites microscopically, including those in the jaw. They concluded that the tumours were all identical and classified them as lymphomas, in other words tumours that arise from white blood cells called lymphocytes. O'Conor and Davies described tumour tissue composed of malignant lymphocytes interspersed with larger, paler staining cells called histiocytes. Under the microscope this pattern resembled a 'starry sky'—a term that is still used to describe the unique appearance of the tumour today.[10] Thereafter the disease became known as the 'lymphoma syndrome' or the 'African lymphoma'. O'Conor and Davies thought that the jaw tumours started growing in bone marrow lymphoid cells inside the jaw bone near developing teeth and spread to other sites from there.

In 1963 another British pathologist, Dennis Wright, began to study the lymphoma syndrome. Wright had been training as a pathologist in England when, in the early 1960s, he knew that he was about to be called up for military service. This he was not keen to do as it would not only separate him from his wife and family but also stall his career in pathology for several years. So when a colleague suggested that he apply for the post of lecturer in pathology at Makerere University, and the army agreed to a stint in Uganda in lieu of National Service, he jumped at the chance. He and his family arrived in Kampala in 1960. At the hospital he found O'Conor enthusiastically working on the lymphoma syndrome while he himself was supposed to be working with Davies on quite a different disease common in Africa at the time—a heart condition called endomyocardial fibrosis. However, the funding for the fibrosis study never materialized and soon after, when both O'Conor and Davies left the hospital, Wright became the resident expert. At this point the lymphoma was thought to be an odd manifestation of other known lymphomas but Wright's work changed all that. He decided to apply some special techniques to pin down the true nature of the tumour cells. For this he had to collect fresh tumour biopsies directly from the operating theatre where Burkitt was working. Then, instead of dropping the material into formalin for permanent preservation as was the usual practice, he made imprints, or touch preparations. These involve gently touching the biopsy on a glass slide thereby depositing some tumour cells onto the slide. The cells could then be stained with dyes, so avoiding the usual fixing, wax embedding, and cutting of the tissue, all of which distort the cell architecture. Using this technique, Wright was able to report that the cell structure of the lymphoma, along with its starry sky appearance, differed from all other lymphomas known at the time.[11] Shortly afterwards, in recognition of its unique characteristics, the tumour was renamed 'Burkitt Lymphoma'.

Burkitt answered the question of how frequently the tumour occurred by scrutinizing hospital case records. He found that the lymphoma was surprisingly common, with an incidence of up to 18 per 100,000 children per year. This made it the most common tumour in children attending the Mulago Hospital, comprising over half of all childhood cancers seen there. It occurred between the ages of 6 months and 14 years, with a peak incidence of between 5 and 6 years. The tumour was seen two to three times more often in boys than girls, was remarkably fast growing, and rapidly fatal. Indeed, Wright and colleagues showed that the number of cells doubled every one to two days,[12] an incredible rate that makes Burkitt Lymphoma the fastest-growing human tumour known.

To find out if the lymphoma syndrome was a new disease, Burkitt visited Mengo mission hospital in Kampala. Founded in 1897 by Sir Albert Cook, a British medical missionary, this was the oldest hospital in East Africa. Cook and his wife Katherine, a nurse, jointly ran the mission hospital for many years, and Burkitt knew that between 1897 and 1944 Cook had kept meticulous medical records of all his patients. Among these he found Cook's descriptions and drawings of jaw tumours in children. The earliest of these dated from 1902, clearly indicating that the disease was not new to the area.

During the early stages of his investigations Burkitt made another highly significant observation. He noticed that, of the children who were referred to Mulago Hospital suffering from the lymphoma, far more lived in the north and east of Uganda than in the south and west. This caught his attention because he would have expected the opposite to be true since the regions to the south and west had larger populations and better transport links with the capital. This fact, along with an assurance from George Oettlé, a visiting pathologist and cancer epidemiologist from Johannesburg, South Africa, that he had never seen a case of Burkitt Lymphoma there, persuaded Burkitt that it must be confined to a specific geographical region. He immediately set about mapping the tumour's distribution in Uganda, reasoning that if such geographical restriction existed, then defining it might help to identify its cause.

Spurred on by the need to investigate further, Burkitt produced leaflets showing a typical case with jaw tumours and a description of the other possible tumour sites. He sent these out to 1,000 government and mission hospitals across Africa together with a questionnaire asking for details of the tumours seen in the area. The many replies he received told him that everywhere where jaw tumours occurred abdominal tumours were also seen, so strengthening the association between the two. They also revealed that the syndrome was common throughout tropical Africa but was not seen in the north or south of the continent. Burkitt was able to map the distribution of the tumour roughly to a region right across Africa between

10 degrees north and 10 degrees south, with a tail running south-wards down the east coast. He referred to this region as the 'lymphoma belt'. Burkitt, who was always at pains to point out that meaningful research need not always be expensive, covered the entire costs of this survey with a government funded grant of just £25 ($75 at the exchange rate of the day). As he said, 'Ideas can more often be turned into dollars than dollars into ideas.'[13]

The results of this small, paper-based survey convinced Burkitt that the lymphoma was a geographically restricted disease, and he set about planning a trip to define the limits of the lymphoma belt more precisely. As luck would have it, he was just wondering how to fund the trip when Sir Harold Himsworth, Director of the Medical Research Council (MRC) in London, visited Kampala and happened to ask Burkitt about his work. The result was a grant of £250 from the MRC towards the cost of the trip. Burkitt used this to cover the travel expenses, principally the purchase of a 1954 Ford station wagon. This was essential for visiting as many medical centres as possible, including remote bush hospitals and missions where lymphoma cases might be seen. With the northern border of the lymphoma belt defined by sparsely inhabited desert, the west and south-western borders by the Atlantic Ocean, and an ongoing revolution in Angola prohibiting exploration to the east, Burkitt aimed to map the southern extent of the eastern border of the belt. He chose two friends and colleagues to accompany him on the trip. First, Ted Williams, a British mission doctor and, importantly, an expert in car maintenance. Williams came from Kuluva Hospital in the remote West Nile region in the north-west corner of Uganda, bordering on the Sudan and the Congo. He and his wife, Muriel, had set up the first mission hospital in the area in the 1940s. We will meet Williams again almost 20 years later when he and Kuluva Hospital played a key role in the large field study examining the link between Epstein-Barr virus infection and the development of Burkitt Lymphoma. The other travelling companion was Cliff Nelson, a Canadian doctor who was in government service in Uganda and later joined Williams at Kuluva.

The three travellers set off on 7 October 1961. The car was laden with food, water, medical supplies, and spare engine parts, and had two spare tyres tied to the roof. Burkitt had meticulously planned every detail in advance and the whole expedition worked like clockwork. During the three months' trip they visited 57 hospitals in eight countries, covering around 10,000 miles (16,090 km) in all. This later became known as 'the long safari' but at the time Burkitt said they regarded it as 'a holiday with a purpose' (see Figure 3a).[14]

Fortunately the jaw tumours were easily recognizable and at each medical centre visited they showed staff photographs of typical cases and asked if they had seen anything similar. The locations of all cases were noted so that when they returned home Burkitt could map the distribution of the disease (Figure 3b). The results were as unexpected as they were dramatic. The tumour appeared to be restricted by altitude. He calculated that at the equator it occurred everywhere except in areas over 5,000 feet (1,524 m) above sea level. However, 1,000 miles south of the equator the tumour was only found below 3,000 feet (914 m), and another 1,000 miles south of that tumours only occurred in the flat coastal regions and river valleys. Thus Burkitt had discovered a tumour that was confined to equatorial Africa and was altitude dependent. With the help of Alexander Haddow, Director of the East African Virus Research Institute at Entebbe, Uganda, he surmised that this bizarre tumour distribution was not due to altitude per se but was caused by temperature sensitivity. Indeed, superimposing a map of the tumour distribution onto a map showing minimum temperatures clearly indicated that it only occurred where the year-round temperature was above 60°F (15°C).

Burkitt made further trips in East Africa, travelling to Rwanda and Burundi, where he found that the association between the tumour incidence and temperature held fast. For the most part this was also true for the information he gained on visits to West African countries, including Nigeria, Ghana, and Zaire. But here he found some anomalies. The highest tumour incidence was recorded in western Nigeria,

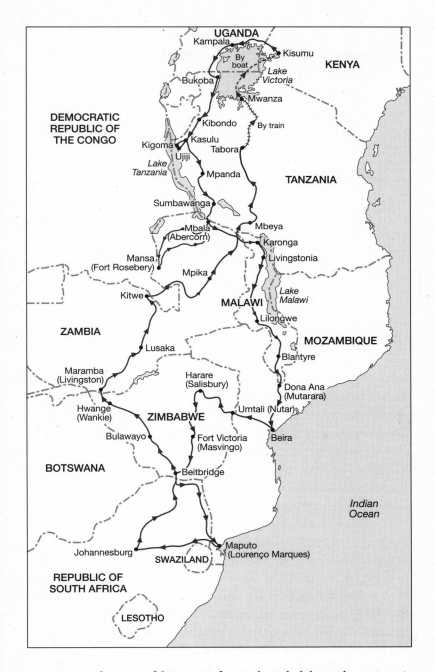

FIGURE 3a The route of the Long Safari, Burkitt's 'holiday with a purpose'.

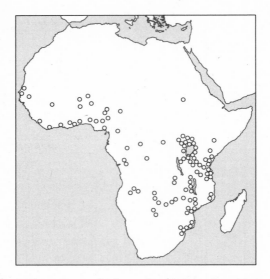

FIGURE 3b Burkitt's map of Africa showing the distribution of Burkitt Lymphoma cases identified during 'the Long Safari'.

but the tumour was not seen at all in Kano in northern Nigeria despite the fact it was a densely populated, low-lying, tropical area. It also had good medical services so it was unlikely that the tumours had been missed by medical staff. Such observations soon uncovered another environmental factor involved in determining tumour distribution— that of rainfall. It turned out that the tumours only occurred where the annual rainfall was above 20 inches (50 cm), thus explaining its absence from the dry savannah of Kano and other similar areas.

Interestingly, when Burkitt later contacted doctors in Papua New Guinea, a group of tropical islands with a climate similar to that of equatorial Africa, he learnt that they also saw children with Burkitt Lymphoma. A review of cases documented by the New Guinea Cancer Registry showed that this was the commonest childhood tumour in the country, with the same age and sex distribution and clinical and pathological features as its African counterpart. Importantly, it was prevalent in the wet, coastal regions but absent in the dry and highland areas, so displaying a dependence on the same environmental factors.[15] Thus Burkitt had clearly demonstrated that the unique geographical restriction of the lymphoma syndrome was explained by its dependence on specific environmental conditions, that is, high annual rainfall and year-round high temperature. Now he and his colleagues set about working out why this should be.

What immediately sprang to mind were the insect-transmitted virus infections, several of which were prevalent in East Africa at the time. One such was yellow fever, which causes fatal liver failure in around 10 per cent of sufferers. Another was O'Nyong-Nyong fever, not generally fatal but a nasty flu-like disease that had recently swept through Uganda infecting almost everyone. Both these diseases are caused by viruses that are carried from one victim to another by mosquitoes. Consequently they are restricted to areas where mosquitoes can breed, that is, regions of high temperature and rainfall. Their distribution maps looked very much like that of Burkitt Lymphoma, strongly suggesting a similar dependence on insect vectors. Thus Burkitt and his colleagues hypothesized that an insect-transmitted virus was the cause of the lymphoma. They thought that this might be a common virus infection, with tumour development as a rare outcome. This theory was supported by the fact that most tumour sufferers were children, the group most likely to be non-immune and therefore susceptible to such an infectious agent.

Intriguingly, Burkitt occasionally saw adults with the lymphoma. These were mainly people who had moved into the lymphoma belt as adults, suggesting that they became infected with a local agent to which they were not immune because they had not been infected during childhood. This was all very plausible, but was it true? Could a *human* tumour really be caused by an insect-transmitted virus?

Several research groups set about trying to answer this question, and Burkitt and his colleagues sent biopsy material to them for virus isolation studies. Among them were American virologist Gilbert Dalldorf, from the Sloan-Kettering Institute in New York, who was based for a time in Nairobi. Dalldorf was well known for the discovery of Coxsackie viruses in 1947, and he isolated a number of different viruses from Burkitt Lymphoma tumours. However, none of these were consistent and none could be directly related to tumour pathogenesis. Around the same time the British Imperial Cancer Research Fund built a research laboratory in Entebbe close to Kampala. This was headed by a Scottish virologist, Thomas Bell, who isolated a reovirus from several Burkitt Lymphoma samples. This virus was referred to as 'respiratory and enteric orphan (reo) virus' because at the time it was not clear that it caused any disease. Some scientists hailed it as the cause of Burkitt Lymphoma but this was never substantiated and the theory was soon abandoned and it was left to others to solve the mystery.

* * *

Once the classic clinical presentation of Burkitt Lymphoma with its characteristic rapidly growing jaw tumours and the unique micro-scopic appearance were widely known, pathologists around the world began to search their archives for similar cases. By the mid 1960s several reports had appeared in the medical literature indicat-ing that Burkitt Lymphoma was not entirely restricted to equatorial Africa and the coastal regions of Papua New Guinea. Isolated cases were seen in the US and Europe but these were very rare, occurring at an incidence of between one and three per million—around 100 times lower than the incidence in the African lymphoma belt.

In 1964 while home on leave in the UK, Wright visited hospitals in several cities to review their cases of childhood lymphoma. To his astonishment he found three cases of Burkitt Lymphoma at the Christie Hospital in Manchester and six at Great Ormond Street Children's Hospital in London. These reports caused great conster-nation at the time as they did not fit with the original hypothesis. In the end Burkitt Lymphoma in the high incidence areas of Africa and Papua New Guinea became known as the 'endemic' form while the rare cases in other sites were labelled the 'sporadic' form of the tumour. Since sporadic tumours were not in areas of high tempera-ture and rainfall, they could not be caused by an insect-vectored virus, a fact that rather weakened Burkitt's theory. Furthermore, at around the same time it became apparent that there were certain large tropical areas, such as parts of South America and Malaysia, where the tumours were not endemic, despite the fact that they fulfilled the environmental conditions for the tumour as described by Burkitt. This was another nail in the coffin of the theory. When none of the viruses then being isolated from samples of the African tumour turned out to be spread by insects, the theory became untenable and was finally abandoned.

Dalldorf and colleagues had published a report on Burkitt Lymphoma in Kenya in 1964 in which they suggested an alternative theory to explain the geographical restriction of the tumour. They thought that malaria infection could be an important factor in the development of Burkitt Lymphoma.[16] After all, the parasite that causes the most severe type of malaria, *Plasmodium falciparum*, is spread by mosquitoes that require high temperature and rainfall for their breeding cycle. They noted that: 'In tropical Africa and New Guinea, the two regions in which this particular form of lymphoma is known to be conspicuously common, an exceptional form of malaria is also prevalent. In both regions the disease is holoendemic [meaning that its transmission persists throughout the year], and repeated infections are nearly universal during the first year of life.' Furthermore *P falciparum* is not found in Malaysia or South America, therefore explaining why Burkitt Lymphoma is not endemic in those countries.

Burkitt and his colleagues now began investigating this theory in Uganda, where they had accurate records on the geographical incidence of Burkitt Lymphoma. Importantly, and quite by coincidence, a large malaria survey had been conducted by the Uganda Malaria Unit between 1963 and 1966. This had examined children in over 100 schools throughout the country and provided detailed information on the regions where holoendemic malaria occurred. Burkitt found a close association between this high intensity of malaria and high tumour incidence. Moreover, the peak age incidence for the tumour coincided with the age at which the children had the highest levels of malaria parasites in their blood.[17] Burkitt's earlier observation of lymphoma in adult migrants into the lymphoma belt could also be explained by this theory as these people were most likely experiencing malaria for the first time, a situation known to cause high levels of blood parasites.

All this information supported a causal relationship between the tumour and holoendemic malaria, which was backed up by two further intriguing, albeit anecdotal, observations. The first of these related to sickle cell anaemia. This is an inherited disorder of the oxygen-carrying molecule, haemoglobin, which is found in red blood cells. In carriers of the sickle cell gene the abnormal haemoglobin causes red cells to adopt a sickle shape rather than being nicely rounded, biconcave discs. Over millennia the sickle cell gene has become remarkably common in tropical Africa because the malaria parasite cannot thrive in sickle cells and thus it protects against fatal malaria. Having two sickle cell genes (one inherited from each parent) can cause severe health problems, whereas inheriting one gene, known as the sickle cell trait, is usually harmless, but is still sufficient to protect against severe malaria. Interstingly, Malcolm Pike, a young South African epidemiologist working at Makerere Medical School, reported on a small study showing that children with sickle cell trait had a lower risk of developing Burkitt Lymphoma than matched control children.[18] The second piece of evidence was that the incidence of Burkitt Lymphoma was found to be low in areas where the environmental conditions were right for the tumour but where intensive malaria eradication programmes had reduced the incidence of malaria. Within Africa this included the island of Zanzibar and the surrounds of Kinshasa, capital of Zaire, and also encompassed some of the small islands of New Guinea.[19] Both these findings supported the hypothesis that severe malaria plays a role in the development of Burkitt Lymphoma. This is still believed to be the case even though, as we shall see, the exact mechanism involved is still not fully understood.

* * *

Like most clinicians who have discovered a new disease, Burkitt was keen to find a treatment that would help Burkitt Lymphoma sufferers, and perhaps even find a cure. Before Burkitt's investigations, surgical removal of tumours in the jaw and other areas was the only treatment. However, once it was appreciated that the disease was virtually always widespread by the time patients came to the hospital, it was obvious that surgery was not appropriate. In theory radiotherapy might have succeeded in shrinking the tumour masses but this was not available in tropical Africa at the time. Burkitt's thoughts therefore turned to chemotherapy. However, anti-cancer drugs were expensive and not affordable in Africa, and thus no one at Mulago Hospital had any experience of using them. But once again luck was on Burkitt's side. In the early 1960s doctors from the Sloan-Kettering Institute for Cancer Research in New York were working at the Kenyatta Hospital in Nairobi with the surgeon Peter Clifford. Among them was a chemo-therapy expert who visited Burkitt in Kampala and was astonished by his first sight of children with the enormous jaw swellings of Burkitt Lymphoma. He gave Burkitt a drug called methotrexate to try, and another doctor, Herbert Oettgen, showed him how to administer it. The first results were very encouraging and so Burkitt persuaded the manufacturer of methotrexate, Lederle Laboratories, to send him the drug free of charge. Burkitt argued that he would be treating a rapidly growing tumour in patients who had not previously been treated with radiotherapy. So, while he would endevour to find the best treatment for his patients, the manufacturers could be sure that any tumour response was entirely due to their drugs. Ethically such a study could only be carried out in a country where radiotherapy was not available, and so Burkitt was able to make similar arrangements with other man-ufacturers who provided the drugs cyclophosphamide and vincristine. He then began to treat the patients, but without any expertise, and with no regulatory authorities to check and approve every drug regi-men, Burkitt proceeded on a trial and error basis. The results were spectacular, leading him to describe himself as 'the most ignorant chemotherapist in the world getting the best results'.[20]

* * *

The work of Burkitt and colleagues in Africa in the six years between 1957 and 1963 was exceptional, and in retrospect was even more remarkable in laying the foundations for the discovery of the first human tumour virus. In those six years Burkitt described a previously unknown clinical entity that came to be known as Burkitt Lymphoma, and uncovered its unique epidemiology. Along with colleagues he later postulated that the tumour was caused by a virus with an insect vector. Although this idea was incorrect, the prediction of a tumour-causing virus eventually proved to be true. Burkitt's description of the unique tumour demographics caught the interest of several researchers, yet Burkitt himself had no formal training in epidemiology and had never worked in a research laboratory—facts of which he was rather proud. His role had been that of a clinician on the ground meticulously observing and recording what he saw. In this case his intense curiosity led to a series of investigations that eventually uncovered the cause of the tumour.

In 1964 Burkitt renounced his career in surgery for a MRC-funded post in Kampala with a remit to investigate the geographical distribution of cancers and other diseases in Africa and beyond. In 1966 he moved back to the UK where this work continued. Then in 1969 Burkitt's natural curiosity led him down a different path in which he was also very influential. He became fascinated with the role of dietary fibre in disease processes, and for the rest of his working life he studied and lectured on this subject, preaching the benefits of a high-fibre, African, diet. In 1976, at the age of 65, Burkitt retired from the MRC, but continued to write, travel, and lecture right up until his death in 1993.

* * *

The search for a virus linked to Burkitt Lymphoma was to develop from another rather unexpected quarter. In 1961, a year before Burkitt undertook his now famous long safari, he had taken a spell of leave in the UK. Here he gave two lectures describing the tumour for the first time outside Africa. One of these was at the Middlesex Hospital in London, where it was attended by the young Anthony Epstein. The far-reaching consequences of this chance meeting are the subject of the next chapter.

2

The Eureka Moment

A nthony Epstein's decision to attend the lecture entitled *The commonest children's cancer in tropical Africa: A hitherto unrecognised syndrome* given by Denis Burkitt at 5.15 p.m. on Wednesday 22 March 1961 in the Courtauld Lecture Theatre at the Middlesex Hospital was a critical one. It not only heralded a turning point in his career but also the advent of human tumour virology. As Burkitt had links with the academic surgery department at the hospital he generally returned there when on leave, usually to give a talk to medical students on the amazing tropical diseases he encountered in East Africa. Normally Epstein would not have been interested but this time the title of the talk hinted at something different. Although he did not know Burkitt, Epstein was sufficiently intrigued to go along to the lecture. Burkitt began by describing the newly discovered tumour with his early observations on its temperature and rainfall dependence, and Epstein recalls that 'after about 10 minutes it was quite obvious to me that this bizarre tumour was unlike anything else. A tumour affected by climate must have a biological cause and I immediately thought of a virus with an insect vector. From that moment in the talk I decided to stop what I was doing and only work on that.' And that is exactly what he did. But this was not just a random decision. It seemed that everything in Epstein's past career had prepared him for this moment. For several years he had been working on a little known cancer-causing virus of chickens, in the belief that lessons learnt would eventually be relevant to human cancer. A human tumour with a possible viral cause was exactly what he was looking for.

Epstein (Figure 4) was born in London in 1921. He attended St Paul's School in London, where he developed a growing interest in biology and eventually decided on a career in medicine. World War II broke out just as he went up to Trinity College, Cambridge, in 1939 and so he completed a shortened 'war degree' course before being hurried to the Middlesex Hospital Medical School in London for clinical training amidst the Blitz. He qualified in 1944 and immediately joined the Royal Army Medical Corps as a lieutenant and later a captain. He served in India from 1945 until 1947 and it was during this time that he realized that his interests lay in laboratory rather than clinical medicine.

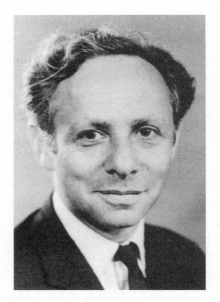

FIGURE 4 Anthony Epstein

Thus it was that after leaving the army Epstein returned to the Middlesex Hospital Medical School to train as a pathologist. He joined the Bland-Sutton Institute, which had a strong tradition of research, and when after nine months of training a research post became available, Epstein was happy to accept it. The subject of the research was Rous sarcoma virus, a virus isolated many years earlier that causes tumours in chickens and named after the American scientist, Peyton Rous, who discovered it. However, this was regarded as a very dubious area of research, perhaps even a dangerous one for a young researcher's career prospects. Epstein recalls that: 'At that time there were perhaps only eight or ten people in the world who were interested in Rous sarcoma virus, [it was] very unfashionable; even a bit eccentric.' Indeed it was *so* unfashionable that Rous, who first published the report describing this 'transmissible agent' in 1911,[21] only received the Nobel Prize for his discovery 55 years later when he was 85 years old. Yet this is perhaps not as surprising as it may at first appear because until the 1930s the real nature of viruses was a mystery. Invisible under a conventional light microscope, they were called 'transmissible agents' and were defined by the fact that they could pass through filters fine enough to retain bacteria and that they would not grow in culture media conventionally used for growing bacteria. At the time most scientists thought that these transmissable agents were probably just very small bacteria, but the invention of the electron microscope in the 1930s revealed the truth. For the first time viruses could be visualized and their structure elucidated. They turned out to be completely unlike bacteria or any other known organism.

Viruses are particles composed of a small piece of genetic material—either DNA or RNA—surrounded by a protective protein coat called a capsid. The particles are inert, meaning that they cannot generate energy, grow, or reproduce on their own. Thus all viruses are parasites that must infect living cells and highjack their protein-making machinery in order to reproduce themselves. Indeed, the fact that virus particles lack all the essential components of living cells raises the question of whether they should be regarded as 'living' at all.

Following the demystification of viruses, many were identified as the cause of common infectious diseases like flu, measles, and small-pox. Flu and measles viruses have RNA genomes while smallpox is a DNA virus, but nevertheless all three viruses infect, reproduce within and then rapidly kill their target cells. This damages the tissues and thereby causes the specific symptoms of the disease. Clearly, if a virus kills the cells it infects it could not cause them to grow into a tumour and so the life cycle of tumour-causing viruses must be very different. We now know that certain RNA and DNA viruses can cause tumours, but identifying them and elucidating the tumourigenic mechanisms they employ took many years.

In the late nineteenth century Louis Pasteur, working in Paris, France, showed that microscopic living organisms in the air could spread infections, while at around the same time Robert Koch from Berlin, Germany, isolated the first bacterium—*Bacillus anthracis*, the cause of anthrax. Thus, between them, these so-called 'fathers of microbiology' showed the 'germ theory' of infection to be true. This soon took hold, replacing the earlier 'miasma theory' that proposed noxious vapours emanating from swamps and rotting material to be the cause of infectious diseases. After this revelation some scientists began to search for microbes that caused cancers. As none were found, the idea soon fell out of favour, but nonetheless, in 1903 a publication from the Pasteur Institute in Paris suggested that cancers may be caused by the invisible 'transmissible agents'.[22] Shortly thereafter, two Danish scientists, Vilhelm Ellerman and Oluf Bang, succeeded in transmitting leukaemia from diseased to healthy chickens with cell-free, tumour extracts that had been passed through filters fine enough to exclude bacteria.[23] Unfortunately, the significance of this experiment was not appreciated at the time because leukaemia was not thought to be a malignant disease. However, just three years later, Rous carried out similar experiments with a chicken sarcoma and was able to induce the same tumours in a series of previously healthy chickens using filtered tumour extracts.

There was little doubt that the chicken sarcoma was a genuine malignant tumour, but despite this the relevance of Rous's work was not appreciated for many years. Rous himself soon gave up working on the sarcoma-inducing agent. Even so, evidence linking certain animal tumours to viruses, variously called 'filterable' or 'sub-microscopic' agents, slowly accumulated. Then 25 years later in 1936 US scientist John Bittner identified a factor in the milk of mice with breast cancer that when ingested by their offspring increased their chances of later developing breast cancer.[24] Bittner cautiously called the factor the 'milk agent' since among the sceptical scientific community at the time calling it a virus would have tended to discredit the work. However, this agent was later shown to be a genuine virus—mouse mammary tumour virus. Occasional reports of such agents appeared over the following two decades, but nevertheless many other attempts to isolate viruses from tumours proved fruitless and so the scientific community continued to doubt the relevance of these odd laboratory findings with animal tumours. In particular, in the absence of any evidence, most scientists rejected the idea that viruses could play a part in the causation of *human* tumours. This was pretty much the situation when Epstein first started work on Rous sarcoma virus in 1948, but he had one huge advantage—access to an electron microscope.

The first electron microscope was built in 1933 by Ernst Ruska, a German physicist who won the Nobel Prize for his invention in 1986. This microscope uses a beam of electrons to illuminate and magnify a specimen. Because electrons have a wavelength around 100,000 times shorter than visible light, the electron microscope can magnify up to 1000 times more than a standard light microscope. The instrument opened up a whole new, sub-cellular world and allowed the structure of viruses to be seen and studied for the first time.

As luck would have it, the Bland-Sutton Institute owned one of the first commercially available electron microscopes, manufactured in the UK by Metropolitan Vickers, and Epstein made good use of it. In 1956 he spent some time working with, and learning from, George Palade at the Rockefeller Institute in New York. Epstein describes Palade as 'a giant in the field…the father of the whole of modern cell biology'. He had developed techniques for examining the internal workings of individual cells using the electron microscope. He then elucidated the structure and function of cellular components such as mitochondria, the cells' energy-generating bodies, and ribosomes, which manufacture proteins. Palade won the Nobel Prize in Physiology or Medicine for this work in 1974.

* * *

When Epstein returned to the Bland-Sutton Institute in 1956 he was well equipped to perform pioneering work on viruses. He was the first to show that Rous sarcoma virus had an RNA genome,[25] and by marking viruses with tiny gold particles he could actually track them as they found their way in and out of cells. So when, in 1961, the chance came to chase a human tumour virus, Epstein was not just receptive but totally inspired. As he says: 'I was so excited by Burkitt's lecture that I actually took the notice off a board, and I still have it!' (Figure 5).

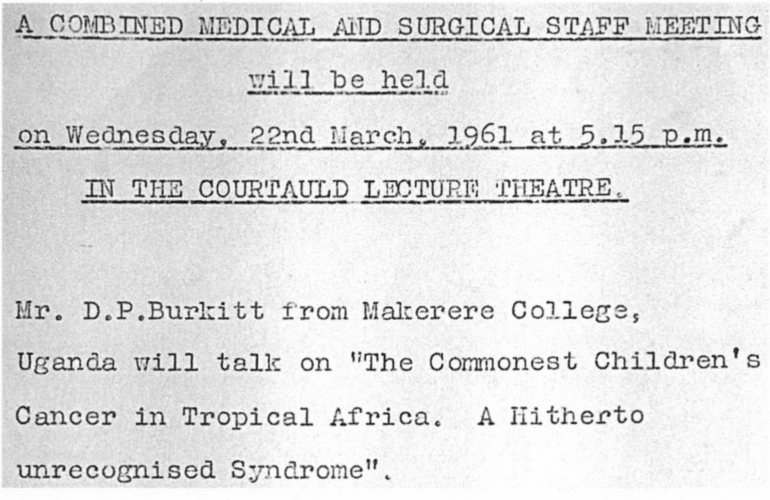

A COMBINED MEDICAL AND SURGICAL STAFF MEETING

will be held

on Wednesday, 22nd March, 1961 at 5.15 p.m.

IN THE COURTAULD LECTURE THEATRE.

Mr. D.P.Burkitt from Makerere College,

Uganda will talk on "The Commonest Children's

Cancer in Tropical Africa. A Hitherto

unrecognised Syndrome".

FIGURE 5 The notice announcing Burkitt's lecture at the Middlesex Hospital in 1961

After the lecture Burkitt and Epstein were formally introduced and sat down to tea together. By the end of the meeting Burkitt had agreed to send tumour specimens to Epstein and Epstein had promised to visit Burkitt at Mulago Hospital to arrange the transportation details. Very soon, fresh Burkitt Lymphoma biopsy specimens were winging their way from Kampala to London on the recently established, overnight jet flights. But although most of the specimens arrived on time and in good condition, things did not go according to plan in the laboratory.

For almost three years all Epstein's attempts to rescue virus from the tumour cells were in vain. Nothing worked, nothing at all. He examined biopsy samples under the electron microscope but saw no viruses. He tried all the traditional virus culture techniques in vogue in the 1960s in the hope of finding a virus. He inoculated Burkitt Lymphoma material onto cells growing in culture medium, onto the membranes of hen's eggs, and into the brains of newborn mice and hamsters, but these also failed to produce a virus. The acute infectious viruses like flu and measles would certainly have grown in these test situations and produced a clearly visible 'plaque' of dead cells. Finally, Epstein recalled that certain chicken tumour viruses would not grow in conventional tests. These viruses only began to reproduce when the malignant cells themselves were grown in culture, a process that somehow activated the latent virus inside them. But, frustratingly, at the time no one had succeeded in growing human lymphocytes—the cell type in Burkitt Lymphoma. Nevertheless, Epstein tried to grow the malignant lymphocytes from tumour samples by all the known methods. He encased them in plasma clots and even floated them on rafts made of teabag paper, but the cells would not grow.

During the summer of 1963 Epstein received a research grant from the US National Institute of Health for $45,000. With this money he was able to employ two research assistants. The first to arrive was a young scientist called Yvonne Barr (Figure 6a). She was a zoology graduate from Trinity College, Dublin, and came to Epstein's laboratory with some experience of cell culture gained from previous posts

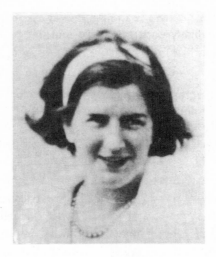

FIGURE 6a Yvonne Barr

at veterinary and medical research establishments in the UK and Canada. She enrolled as a graduate student and set about tending the Burkitt Lymphoma cell cultures. She recalls that when the precious biopsies arrived in the laboratory she would set them up in culture with just two millilitres of growth medium in tiny glass insulin bottles. But none of the cultures would grow; a situation that must have been very frustrating.

Eventually, with so many negative results Epstein felt that his career was on the line. He had put all his eggs into one basket and was banking on a positive result. The same position today would be highly risky if not suicidal to one's career in science, and Epstein now admits that even then the situation was 'extremely alarming…scary'. But when asked if he ever thought that he was mistaken in his hunch that Burkitt Lymphoma was caused by a virus he replies with conviction 'never'. And to an enquiry as to what caused the up-turn in his fortunes he promptly answers 'fog'.

On the morning of Friday 5 December 1963 a biopsy sample taken from the upper jaw of a 9-year-old girl with Burkitt Lymphoma was expected to arrive from Kampala. But, because Heathrow airport was fog-bound, all incoming flights were diverted to Manchester, some 200 miles away. The sample eventually arrived in the laboratory in the late afternoon just as everyone was packing up and heading home for the weekend. The biopsy was in a bottle of the usual transport medium composed of a salt solution and guinea pig serum, but instead of being clear the fluid was cloudy. This suggested that the prolonged journey had allowed bacteria to grow in the fluid. Such contaminated samples would normally be discarded, but despite the late hour Epstein decided to examine the fluid under a light microscope. He was 'absolutely astonished to see not bacteria seething away but a huge number of viable, free floating tumour cells that had been shaken off from the edges of the biopsy in the journey'.

Epstein was immediately reminded of cells he had seen the previous summer when he visited a team of scientists at Yale University Medical School, Newhaven, US. They had been studying lymphomas in mice and had only succeeded in growing the tumour cells by starting with a suspension of free-floating cells, rather than the more traditional solid tumour fragments. Until that time all successful growth of cells in culture involved the cells sticking to a glass surface for support. But on that day, for the first time, Epstein decided to put the free-floating Burkitt tumour cells into a suspension culture, just in case it would make a difference.

Barr also remembers that this, the 26th biopsy to arrive from Uganda, was different from all the others. After 16 days in culture, just before Christmas, there was an encouraging sign in one of the culture bottles. The fluid had changed colour—a sure indication that the cells had begun to grow. By the 26th day (New Year's Eve 1963) there were enough cells to divide the culture into two, and by day 43 the growing cells were transferred to larger bottles. Barr recalls that when she examined the culture under a light microscope, 'the cells glistened—a sign of life. They were round. They were lymphoblasts—a cell type that little was known about...What excitement! The cells grew up and the first Burkitt's Lymphoma derived cell line christened EB1, E for Epstein, B for Barr, was established.'

The cells grew continuously, forming the immortal cell line, EB1, which is still growing to this day. This represented the first successful long-term culture of a human lymphoma of any kind, and Epstein and Barr rushed to publish reports describing the cell line and their technique for growing the cells.[26, 27] As it happened, unknown to Epstein and Barr, short-term Burkitt Lymphoma cell cultures were being set up in Nigeria by Robert Pulvertaft, a pathologist from the Westminster Medical School in London, who in 1964 was a visiting professor at the University of Ibadan.[28] He was studying the appearance of the fresh tumour cells and, subsequently, two Burkitt Lymphoma cell lines grew out. These cell lines, called Raji and Jijoye after tumours from children of the same names, were later grown, characterized and distributed worldwide by others.[29] They have since been used in some key experiments; we will come across them again in chapter 3. Importantly, Pulvertaft's publication describing the cultured Burkitt Lymphoma cells meant that EB1 was not just a one-off, and that given the right culture conditions Burkitt Lymphoma cells really did have the unique capacity to grow continuously in culture. Indeed, over the coming months Epstein and Barr established more cell lines from Burkitt tumour biopsies, labelling them EB2, EB3, and so on. The trick was to detach the cells from the tumour fragments and grow them in suspension culture, an entirely new technique and one that allowed the cells to be propagated ad infinitum.

The second research assistant Epstein employed in 1963 was Bert Achong (Figure 6b). He was a graduate of University College Dublin but he grew up in Port of Spain, Trinidad, where he was educated at St Mary's Catholic College. From there he won a scholarship to study medicine in Ireland, qualifying as a doctor in 1953. In 1955 he moved to London to train as a pathologist, and it was late in 1963 when he joined Epstein's research team. According to Achong he was offered the choice of a project using the electron microscope to study the ultra-structure of Burkitt Lymphoma cells or a project on liver

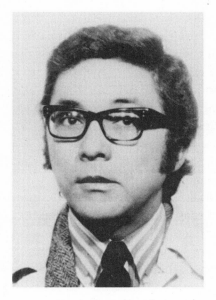

FIGURE 6b Bert Achong

cancer. Knowing nothing about either subject he decided on the Burkitt Lymphoma project by the toss of a coin!

Shortly after Achong joined the group the EB1 cell line became the focus of attention. It promised to provide a ready source of tumour cells in which to search for a virus, but, depressingly the results were just as had been seen with the biopsy material. All conventional tests for rescuing a virus from the cultured cells were negative. There was just one thing left to try—electron microscopy. And so as soon as sufficient EB1 cells were available they were prepared for this technique. At the time this technique was definitely *not* an accepted way to hunt for new viruses. Many scientists even regarded the images it generated, including those of putative viruses, as nothing more than artefacts produced by the preparation procedures. They certainly did not believe that the structural characteristics of different virus families could be distinguished by this means. Despite this, Epstein was sure that electron microscopy was the way to go.

Finally, on 24 February 1964, the EB1 cells were ready to be examined under the Institute's electron microscope, by now a much more powerful Philips 200 EM machine. As Epstein entered the dark room that housed the electron microscope he had no idea how easy the task of virus hunting would be. In the very first grid square he looked at he saw something amazing—'a cell filled with herpesvirus!' He recalls that 'I was so amazed and euphoric that I was terrified that the specimen would burn up in the electron beam. So I switched off and walked round the block without a coat in the snow. By the time I had calmed down I came back and took pictures.'

When asked if he had any doubt about what he had seen he replies 'No, no doubt at all, it was obvious. I knew what I was looking at.'

Epstein was instantly convinced that the viruses he saw in EB1 cells were herpesviruses (Figure 7), but unfortunately this conviction was not shared by the scientific community at large. Epstein, Achong, and Barr first published their discovery in *The Lancet* on 28 March 1964.[30] In the report they described the virus particles they had seen in a few of the cultured Burkitt Lymphoma cells—actually in around 1 per cent of the cells, which just shows how lucky Epstein had been to see viruses in the first grid he examined. The authors reasoned that the virus in EB1 cells was structurally similar to herpes simplex virus and was therefore a herpesvirus. They noted that the particles were consistently smaller in size than herpes simplex virus, suggesting, but not proving, that it was a different type of herpesvirus. However, at this stage they were careful not to claim this as a new discovery or that the virus they saw was related to the cause of Burkitt Lymphoma. Even so the report was greeted with a great deal of disbelief—viruses present in a small minority of cells in the cell line suggested to most scientists that they represented an infection with a contaminating virus. It took many years of hard work to provide convincing evidence that, not only was the virus an entirely new human herpesvirus, but also that it was causally related to Burkitt Lymphoma.

The herpesvirus family has literally hundreds of members. Most vertebrates, and even some invertebrates, carry their own particular

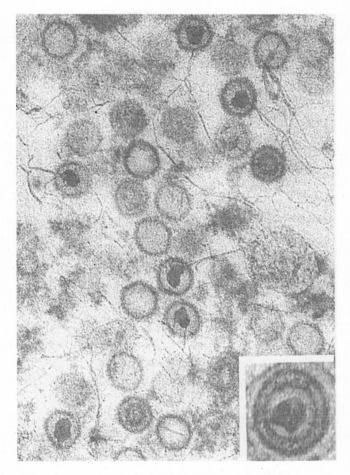

FIGURE 7 Electronmicrograph of thin sectioned EBV. Numerous immature virus particles are seen within a virus-producing cell. Inset, a single mature virus particle.

family members, and to date eight human herpesviruses have been discovered. However, in 1964 only three of these were known—herpes simplex, the cold sore virus; varicella zoster, the chicken pox virus; and the salivary gland virus now known as cytomegalovirus. Herpesviruses are large DNA viruses with a characteristic shape and size, being icosahedral (20-sided) and 70–100 microns in diameter (Figure 7). This is how Epstein was so sure that he had seen herpesviruses in the EB1 cells he examined under the electron microscope. However, human herpesviruses infect virtually everyone, usually gaining access to the body during childhood without causing any illness. Then, like a silent lodger, they hide in particular types of cells for a whole lifetime. This silent, or latent, infection may reactivate to cause disease, as in recurrent episodes of cold sores and genital ulcers caused by herpes simplex, or shingles caused by varicella zoster virus often many years after an attack of chickenpox. So from the image of the virus Epstein saw under the electron microscope it was not possible for him to tell whether he was looking at one of these common, resident herpesviruses or at a completely 'new' virus.

Epstein and his team purified the virus from EB1 cells and set about testing its biological activity. Again they used all the routine virology tests of the day—growth in cultured cell lines, in hens' eggs, and in newborn mice. They repeated the tests endlessly, but every time the results were totally negative—the virus simply would not grow. So either this was a completely new virus that was not recognized by routine tests or, more worryingly, the test results were negative because Epstein and his team were killing the virus during the preparation procedures. Epstein remembers, 'That's when the doubt came—what on earth were we doing to inactivate this virus?'

Left with a virus that was just an image under the electron microscope, Epstein eventually decided that they needed expert help—someone who could repeat the tests and either confirm the results or uncover an error in their processing procedure. He approached two British virologists but neither was interested in investigating what they probably did not believe was a virus at all. So Epstein approached his colleagues and friends, Werner and Gertrude Henle, a husband and wife team of virologists working at the Children's Hospital in Philadelphia, US. We will meet the Henles and their work on the virus again in chapter 3, but in the 1960s they jointly ran one of the largest diagnostic and research virology laboratories in the US.

Epstein had visited their laboratory on his first trip to the US in 1956 and also on several subsequent occasions, and now they agreed to carry out tests on the 'new' virus. So began a long and fruitful collaboration.

Epstein sent the Henles Burkitt Lymphoma cell lines EB1 and EB2 and Gertrude Henle repeated the attempts to grow the virus that had given Epstein's team such frustratingly negative results. The results were again negative, but for once negative results were good news. They suggested that the virus was really inactive in routine tests and that Epstein and colleagues had not unwittingly killed it during purification. This was quite unlike the other known herpesviruses—herpes simplex, varicella zoster, and cyotmegalo- viruses—they would certainly have grown in some or all of these tests. Therefore the virus in cultured Burkitt Lymphoma cells was unique—it was indeed a 'new' human herpesvirus!

Epstein, Achong, Barr, and Gertrude Henle jointly reported their findings confirming the discovery of the new human herpesvirus in 1965.[31] They initially referred to it as the 'herpes-like agent from Burkitt Lymphoma', but the Henles later christened it EBV for Epstein-Barr Virus after the series of 'EB' cell lines Epstein had sent them.

Once they had identified the unique virus in Burkitt Lymphoma cells the next obvious question was: is EBV the cause of Burkitt Lymphoma? Or, alternatively, is it just a passenger virus that likes to grow in Burkitt Lymphoma cells?

* * *

The issue of causality must have had a particular resonance for Werner Henle because of an interesting family connection. In the mid 1900s a German anatomist, Jacob Henle, grandfather to Werner Henle, began to put together criteria for establishing a causal link between a microbe and a specific disease. This was further developed by his pupil, the famous Robert Koch, and the set of criteria that evolved, variously called the Koch, or Henle-Koch, postulates, lists the principles that must be fulfilled before claiming that a microbe is the cause of a specific disease. Initially these were as follows:

- The microbe occurs in every case of the disease in question and can account for the pathological changes and clinical course of the disease.
- The microbe occurs in no other disease
- After being isolated and grown in culture the microbe can reproduce the disease in an experimental animal.

These postulates referred primarily to bacteria and even Koch himself admitted that the criteria could not all be met for every bacterial infection. Certain bacteria proved difficult to isolate from all cases of the disease in question: some were found in people with no symptoms and others were very difficult to grow in the laboratory. Also, suitable animal models were not always available and it was clearly not ethical to inject a microbe suspected of causing a human disease into healthy human subjects. These problems were compounded after the discovery of viruses since they are often more difficult to isolate and grow in culture. Thus over the years the principles have been revised and other criteria have been added. In particular, testing for antibodies can identify those who have been infected by a specific microbe. This test is a lot easier than virus isolation and has the advantage of being amenable for use in large-scale surveys. Such evidence was to become instrumental in linking EBV to Burkitt Lymphoma.

To fulfil Koch's revised postulates, ideally Epstein and colleagues had to show that EBV was present in all Burkitt Lymphoma tumours; that all children with Burkitt Lymphoma had antibodies to EBV; that EBV could infect normal lymphocytes and 'transform' them into malignant cells; and that EBV caused lymphoma in a suitable animal model. This was no small order and it took many research groups several decades to satisfy these criteria. The quest had its highs and lows: some of the criteria were straightforward to demonstrate while investigation of others uncovered unforeseen complexities that only led to further questions. The studies that provided the answers are described in the following chapters.

* * *

By 1966 Barr had completed her doctoral studies and gained a PhD from the University of London. Following her three years at the Bland-Sutton Institute, Barr married and emigrated to Melbourne, Australia, where she spent 20 years teaching science and maths in state schools. She retired in 1993 and, at the time of writing still lives in Victoria.

Achong was awarded an MD by University College, Dublin, for his work on the fine structure of Burkitt Lymphoma cells in 1965. He continued to work with Epstein, moving with him to the Department of Pathology at the University of Bristol in 1968. In addition to working on EBV he lectured on cellular pathology using his unique combination of charm and erudition to enthral generations of grateful students. He retired in 1985 and died in London in 1996.

Epstein devoted the rest of his working life to EBV research, in particular to the production of a vaccine. If successful, he argued, this would not only prevent deaths from EBV associated diseases but also provide incontrovertible proof that the virus caused those diseases.

3

Convincing the Sceptics

Werner Henle and Gertrude Szpingier met in the early 1930s when they were both studying medicine at the University in Heidelberg, Germany. Gertrude, who was always called Brigitte by family and friends, was born in Mannheim in Germany. Werner had also been born and brought up in Germany. However, his famous grandfather, Jacob Henle, was Jewish. In 1930s Germany with the Nazis on the rise, this Jewish connection was enough to blight Werner's career and perhaps even threaten his life. Consequently, like so many Jewish doctors of his generation, he fled Germany soon after he qualified as a doctor. He sailed to the US in 1934 and Gertrude followed him as soon as she graduated in 1937. They married on the day of her arrival in New York and then worked together for over 40 years jointly running the Virus Diagnostic Laboratory at the Children's Hospital of Philadelphia (Figure 8).

The Henles' laboratory was well established as one of the largest and most respected in the US by 1965 when Epstein proposed a collaboration on the virus he had isolated from Burkitt Lymphoma cells. Until that time the Henles had worked mainly on flu and mumps vaccines but they both jumped at the chance to investigate a potential human tumour virus. They immediately dropped all other

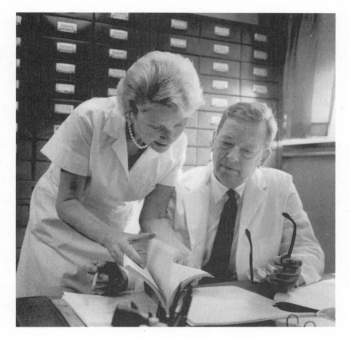

FIGURE 8 Gertrude and Werner Henle

research to dedicate their efforts to EBV, and, as we shall see, in doing so they made some hugely important discoveries.

When the Henles found that the virus did not perform like any known herpesvirus in the routine tests running in their diagnostic laboratory they were convinced that this was a new member of the herpes virus family. However, this did not prove that the virus was the cause of Burkitt Lymphoma, and, just like Epstein in the UK, for a while the Henles faced criticism from some famous US scientists who did not believe that viruses could cause human tumours. In particular, those working on animal RNA tumour viruses like Rous sarcoma virus, mouse mammary tumour virus, and mouse leukaemia virus, at the US National Cancer Institute in Maryland could not accept that a DNA herpesvirus could be tumourigenic. So now it was important to find out more, and initially the Henles concentrated on looking at who was infected with the new virus.

This involved setting up a test to screen people for past infection with EBV by detecting serum antibodies directed against virus proteins. The Henles used EB1 cells as targets in the test since they knew that Epstein had seen virus particles in around 1 per cent of these cells. The idea was that when a test serum containing specific antibodies to EBV was exposed to EB1 cells the antibodies would recognize and stick to the few virus-containing cells. Then the antibody-coated cells could be lit up by adding a fluorescent reagent that detected the antibody molecules stuck to the cells. Sure enough, when they tested a serum sample from a Burkitt Lymphoma patient and then looked at the cells under a microscope fitted with an ultraviolet light source, around 1 per cent of the cells glowed with beautiful apple green flourescence. The Henles must have been delighted—and even more so when they tested 17 further sera from Burkitt Lymphoma patients and all reacted in the same way. So all these Burkitt Lymphoma patients had been infected by EBV—a step in the right direction for linking the virus to the tumour.

But then came the first surprise. When the Henles tested blood samples from American adults, over 90 per cent were also EBV antibody positive, indicating a past or present infection. It did not make any difference whether they were healthy or suffering from various forms of cancer, almost all were positive. Thirty per cent of hospitalized American children were also EBV positive regardless of any illness they had. So the virus was obviously very common in the US.[32] Looking further afield they soon discovered evidence of a worldwide distribution—even those living in isolated communities were infected, including members of Amazonian tribes and inhabitants of remote islands—so EBV was ubiquitous. This was puzzling if the virus was specifically linked to Burkitt Lymphoma: in fact the only difference between those with Burkitt Lymphoma and those without was that the former consistently had higher levels of EBV antibodies in their blood than the latter.

Among children in the US, the Henles found that the timing of first (primary) EBV infection was similar to that seen for common infections such as flu and measles viruses. The percentage of children with antibodies gradually increased with age until reaching the high adult levels. This suggested that EBV was often acquired in childhood and might even be the cause of a common childhood illness, but despite extensive testing, no connection to any particular illness could be found. The Henles published these results in 1966. Once again they faced criticism from RNA tumour virologists who suggested that their antibody test was not specific—perhaps it was just picking up dead cells in the EB1 culture.

* * *

On their regular visits to Heidelberg in the 1960s the Henles took the opportunity to interview young medical graduates who might be interested in working in the US. Two such candidates were Harald zur Hausen and Volker Diehl, both of whom later were to become famous for their own work in the fields of tumour virology and haematology/oncology respectively. They were interviewed and both were subsequently offered research posts to work on a new virus—EBV.

Thus by 1966 the Henles had two new medical researchers in their team—the first to work specifically on EBV. Both zur Hausen and Diehl remember the Henles with affection. Diehl recalls 'a very kind couple…intelligent and sophisticated', and while Werner was 'a gentleman, very quiet and relaxed, a thinker', Gertrude was 'mostly talking, very active and always had new ideas'. Perhaps because of their very different personalities, the Henle husband and wife team worked well and the lasting partnership produced several dramatic breakthroughs. On a day–to-day basis Gertrude ran the laboratory and supervised the staff. She was competitive, impatient for results, and mercurial—as Diehl recalls, 'Harald and I joked about it because every day she had 1000 new ideas!'

Zur Hausen recalls that he had known nothing about EBV when he met the Henles in Heidelberg and Gertrude overwhelmed him with information about the new virus. However, by the time he began work in Philadelphia in January 1966 he had done his home-work and was excited to be working on the EBV project. This was particularly so because, despite the scepticism prevalent at the time, even as a medical student zur Hausen had thought that viruses could be involved in human cancers. For three years after graduating zur Hausen worked on adenovirus, a DNA virus that had been found to cause tumours in laboratory animals, at the Dusseldorf Institute of Microbiology. On arrival in the US he was ready for the challenge of discovering more about a potential human tumour virus, although he never completely gave up his interest in adenoviruses.

Given the criticism they had received regarding their EBV anti-body test, the Henles were obviously keen to show that the EB1 cells that lit up in the test did indeed contain virus particles. Thus zur Hausen was persuaded to find a way of isolating individual fluorescing cells and then to examine them for viruses under the electron microscope. After a few teething problems he managed to show that the fluorescing cells did indeed contain EBV particles and this, denoting that the antibody test was specific, was a welcome result for the Henles. The actual virus protein (antigen) that antibodies bound to in this test was not identified for some time but since the test only picked up cells containing maturing virus particles (capsids), it became known as the virus capsid antigen test.

Having completed this piece of work there were other research problems that zur Hausen found more enticing. While some Burkitt Lymphoma cell lines like EB1 contained a few cells that produced virus particles, others, like the Raji cell line established by Pulvertaft (see chapter 2) seemed to produce no virus and did not react at all in the Henles' antibody test. So the question that interested zur Hausen was why most or all of the cells in Burkitt Lymphoma cell lines showed no sign of virus production. He often discussed this problem with Werner Henle and they came up with two alternative explanations. On one hand, the virus genome might be present in all the cells in the culture but either none of these cells could support the production of new virus particles or, at any one time only a few could do so, and they would die in the process. If true, then all tumour cells must carry the virus genome as a latent (silent) infection that was compatible with continued growth of the cell, and perhaps could even stimulate tumour outgrowth. On the other hand, the virus might be present as a low-level contaminating infection in the cultures, infecting only a very small number of cells at any one time. The infected cells would die producing new virus particles that were slowly passed on to a few neighbouring cells and from them to a few more cells, and so on. In this scenario the Raji cell line would not be infected at all or else the infection must be so sparse that it was undetectable in the fluorescence test.

While the first suggestion would implicate the virus in actually *inducing* continuous growth of the cells and thus support its role in tumour production, the second relegated the virus to the status of a mere passenger whose presence had nothing to do with tumour growth. At the time zur Hausen was inclined towards the former explanation; the more experienced Werner Henle feared the latter.

Zur Hausen realized that if EBV established a latent infection in Burkitt Lymphoma cells, without expressing the structural proteins required for virus production, then the best way to find it was by detecting its DNA genome. This would need molecular biological techniques that were only just being developed at the time and were not available in the Henles' laboratory. He proposed to learn these techniques, apply them to detecting adenovirus DNA in adenovirus-infected cells in the first instance and then return to EBV to see if he could detect its DNA in Burkitt Lymphoma cell lines. While Werner was prepared to go along with this plan, Gertrude was not. It was her habit to provide researchers with a protocol each morning that she expected them to follow. Zur Hausen remembers that when he ignored these protocols 'she became more and more impatient with me'. Their relationship only improved six months later when he had some interesting results, albeit from some adenovirus experiments. Eventually the goal finding EBV DNA in Burkitt Lymphoma cells was realized but that lay some way in the future.

* * *

When Diehl arrived in Philadelphia to work with the Henles in June 1966 he was somewhat dismayed to find that the laboratory was 'dark, a little bit crumby, with small rooms, and in the middle of the slums of Philadelphia'. He recalls: 'I had a beautiful little Volkswagen. I was very proud of it…when I parked it in front of the building in South Philadelphia it was broken into nearly every night!'

Despite his initial reservations Diehl got on well with the Henles and enjoyed the time he spent working in their laboratory. First he set about tackling the important question of whether, in the laboratory, EBV had the properties expected of a tumour virus. In particular, could EBV infection of normal human lymphocytes (which do not grow in culture) transform them into rapidly growing cell lines akin to those derived from Burkitt Lymphoma biopsy cells? Unfortunately, even the best virus-producing line around at the time, Jijoye, originally established by Pulvertaft (see chapter 2), only made tiny amounts of virus, and so purifying enough for these experiments was very difficult. To circumvent this problem, Diehl and Werner Henle devised an ingenious plan. First they hit Jijoye cells with a blast of X-rays that stopped the cells growing and dividing but did not immediately kill them. Thus the cells remained alive in the culture for a week or so and continued to produce virus particles. They then mixed these X-irradiated cells with cord blood lymphocytes—that is lymphocytes purified from blood taken from a vein in the portion of an umbilical cord left attached to the placenta after the birth of a baby. This may seem a very odd choice for a source of lymphocytes, but it was to ensure that the cells came from someone (a newborn baby) who had definitely not already been infected with EBV. They carefully chose cord blood samples from babies of the opposite sex to that of the irradiated Burkitt cells they were using, and then they waited to see what would happen. As a control they also included similar cultures where the Jijoye cells were replaced with the non-virus-producing Burkitt cell line, Raji. Their hope was that virus produced by the X-irradiated Jijoye cells would infect the normal cord blood lymphocytes in the culture and induce them to grow, while all the cells in cultures containing X-irradiated Raji cells would die. Diehl studiously observed the cultures every day for the next two or three months, but nothing seemed to be happening. Then one night when for some reason he was in the laboratory at two o'clock in the morning he noticed that cells were beginning to grow in the cultures containing Jijoye cells. He promptly phoned Werner Henle. He recalls that he 'shook him out of bed and said, "Werner they grew!" We got extremely excited!'

Gratifyingly, no cells grew in the cultures containing Raji cells while growth appeared in several of the Jijoye-containing cultures. The finding was reproducible but still before publishing this revelation the team had to be sure that it was indeed the cord blood lymphocytes and not the Burkitt Lymphoma cells that were growing in the Jijoye cultures. With the carefully organized sex mismatch between the Burkitt and cord blood cells this was easy. All they had to do was examine the sex chromosomes of the growing cells. When they turned out to be the sex of the cord blood lymphocytes they knew for certain that EBV was a transforming virus. So in 1967 the Henle group was the first to show that EBV infection of normal human lymphocytes could convert them from non-dividing cells into continuously growing cell lines—another crucial step towards proving that EBV was a tumour virus.[33]

By coincidence, at the same time as Diehl was making these discoveries, on the other side of the world John Pope, a virologist from the Queensland Institute for Medical Research in Brisbane, Australia, was performing very similar experiments.[34] He first became interested in EBV when he grew cell lines from Burkitt Lymphoma biopsies that he obtained from nearby New Guinea. He found that, like their African counterparts, these cell lines contained a few virus-producing cells. Simultaneously, he also found virus particles in cell lines that he grew from the blood of patients with leukaemia. In this case the cell lines were clearly not derived from the leukaemia cells. In fact he was observing 'spontaneous transformation'—the occasional growth of EBV-transformed cells in cultures set up from the blood of anyone, healthy or not, who has been infected with EBV and continues to carry the virus. One such cell line produced enough virus for Pope to purify, and he showed that this virus also transformed cord blood cells into continuously growing cell lines much as Henle and Diehl's irradiated Jijoye cells had done. Thus Pope's experiments corroborated and extended the results of the Henle group.

When these studies on lymphocyte transformation were published in 1968, the word 'lymphocyte' was thought to describe a single cell type, since they all looked alike under the light microscope. But immunologists were already beginning to develop markers to distinguish between subsets of lymphocytes with different functions within the immune system. We now know that one subset, the B lymphocytes, is the group that produces antibodies (or immunoglobulins) against foreign proteins. Another broad subset, the T lymphocytes, provide help to B lymphocytes in that role and also give rise to so-called 'killer T cells' that control virus infections by killing infected cells. Studies in the early 1970s showed that EBV specifically attaches to, and infects, only cells of the B lymphocyte subset.[35] This is possible because a unique protein called gp 340/350 that is part of the virus envelope binds to a cell surface protein specific to B lymphocytes called CD21.[36] Accordingly, the cell lines that arose from EBV-infected cord blood cell cultures were identified as virus-transformed B lymphocytes, and Burkitt Lymphoma was likewise shown to be a B lymphocyte-derived tumour. The parallels between EBV's behaviour in the laboratory and its association with a lymphoma now seemed stronger than ever.

* * *

Another burning question often discussed by the Henles' group at the time concerned the kind of illness EBV—a potential tumour virus—might cause in the Western world. Soon after the first description of Burkitt Lymphoma and its unique geographical distribution it was suggested that the tumour might be related to acute lymphoblastic leukaemia.[37] This was because both malignancies target the same cells—lymphocytes—and both occur mainly in children. Crucially, the geographical distributions of the two diseases were mutually exclusive. While Burkitt Lymphoma was very common in the tropics, acute childhood leukaemia was extremely rare. Exactly the opposite was true in the Western world, giving rise to the theory that the two diseases could represent different manifestations of the same infection. The Henles tested blood samples from people with all manner of infectious diseases and tumours, including children with acute lymphoblastic leukaemia, but none gave the hoped-for result. They were looking for diseases with 100 per cent EBV positivity and high antibody levels such as those seen in Burkitt Lymphoma, or ideally a *seroconversion*. This means that a person who was EBV antibody negative before the onset of a specific disease developed these antibodies during the illness. This would indicate primary EBV infection as the cause of the disease, but the search was proving fruitless; it was like looking for a needle in a haystack. That is until one memorable day in 1967 when, quite by chance, the breakthrough came.

On 10 August a technician called Elaine Hutkin who worked in the Henles' laboratory with Diehl was unwell and did not show up for work. After she had been absent for a few days Gertrude Henle became impatient and insisted that she came to the laboratory. Diehl called her up and although at first she said she was too sick to come she was eventually persuaded to make an appearance. Sure enough, when she turned up on the 16 August she was obviously very unwell. Diehl examined her and found that she had a fever, enlarged lymph glands (lymphadenopathy) and spleen (splenomegaly) and aggressive tonsillitis. He took a blood sample from her for diagnostic tests and sent her home to recover. But already he had an idea what she was suffering from—she had all the symptoms of infectious mononucleosis, also called glandular fever.

* * *

Most people with infectious mononucleosis go to the doctor complaining of a sore throat, fever, and enlarged lymph glands. The illness usually lasts around 10 to 14 days and full recovery is the rule. However, on occasions the symptoms can be severe enough to require hospital admission, generally because of liver damage or difficulty in swallowing and breathing due to severe inflammation of the throat. Also, patients often experience overwhelming fatigue that in some cases may extend the illness for up to six months, causing major loss of work time. Infectious mononucleosis most often occurs between the ages of 15 and 25 years and is particularly common among college and university students.

Infectious mononucleosis was first described by Nil Filatov, a Russian paediatrician, in 1885, and independently by Emil Pfeiffer, a German physician, in 1889. The name 'infectious mononucleosis' was first coined in 1920 when distinctive changes in the blood were first noted. Early in the disease there is a dramatic increase of cells in the blood that were originally called 'atypical mononuclear cells', now known to be large, activated lymphocytes. This is a constant feature of the disease and often helps to distinguish it from other causes of severe sore throat. However, on occasions the numbers of these cells can be so high that, in the past, infectious mononucleosis was sometimes misdiagnosed as acute leukaemia.

A diagnostic test for the disease called the 'heterophil antibody test' was devised in 1932. In those days it was a long, laborious test to perform but it nevertheless allowed most cases of the disease to be diagnosed. Though infectious mononucleosis seemed to be caused by a virus, the identity of that virus and its method of spread remained an enigma. Unlike the typical airborne epidemic viruses, measles and chickenpox, infectious mononucleosis was rarely seen in children and did not cause major outbreaks. Furthermore, although it was particularly common among students, sufferers virtually never reported contact with a case of the disease, and there was no evidence of spread between those sharing a bedroom or dormitory. Hospitalized cases were nursed in an open ward without fear of cross infection.

This all pointed to a non-airborne causative agent, and attempts were made to find it by reproducing the disease in animals. When transferring gargle throat washings, blood, or lymph gland cells from infectious mononucleosis patients to monkeys, rabbits, guinea pigs and mice all failed, experimenters turned to using human volunteers. Several studies carried out in during the 1940s, 1950s, and early 1960s used consenting medical students as guinea pigs, experiments that would be unthinkable today. Blood from patients was injected, throat gargle washings were sprayed into the nose and throat or swallowed, and even faecal preparations were introduced into the stomach via a tube. But all to no avail. Only when large quantities of blood (250–400 ml) were transferred to a volunteer from an acutely ill patient did the symptoms of infectious mononucleosis occasionally appear in the recipient. These findings were backed up by transmission via a blood transfusion which was eventually accomplished, albeit unwittingly, in 1951. In this case the blood came from a donor who developed infectious mononucleosis one week after donating the blood. The recipient of the blood developed the typical symptoms 21 days later. Although this suggested that the infectious agent was present in the blood at a very early stage in the disease, clearly transmission via blood seemed very unlikely to be the agent's natural route of spread.[38]

In 1955 Colonel Robert J Hoagland, Chief of Medicine at 139th Station Hospital in New York, postulated that the infectious mononucleosis agent was spread by 'intimate oral contact which permits a transfer of saliva'.[39] This theory resulted from six years' observation of the disease at the US Military Academy and much searching out and reading of reported cases. He was particularly taken by the story of a young man in whom he diagnosed the disease. In a scenario reminiscent of the classic film *Brief Encounter*, 49 days before his illness the man had spent 12 hours on a train with a female medical student. They had not met before or since this encounter, but during the journey they had kissed frequently 'in a way that allowed mingling of saliva'. On contacting her at the time of the young man's illness it transpired that she too had been in hospital, also suffering from infectious mononucleosis.

From his collected case histories Hoagland suggested that the incubation period for infectious mononucleosis was between 33 and 49 days. Among his many cases he cites the story of three sailors who came down with infectious mononucleosis within a week of each other while aboard a destroyer. Despite the cramped living, working and sleeping conditions aboard ship, the disease spread no further. The sailors' last visit ashore had been five weeks previously when, Hoagland surmised, they had picked up the infectious agent through 'intimate oral contact'. Thus infectious mononucleosis was dubbed 'the kissing disease'.

* * *

Now back to Philadelphia in August 1967 where Hutkin's blood samples sent for diagnostic testing showed many atypical mononuclear cells and her heterophil antibody test was positive, so she did indeed have infectious mononucleosis. But there was more. As in many virology laboratories at the time, blood was regularly taken from the Henles' staff for use as controls in routine tests. Hutkin's serum had previously been tested for EBV antibodies on several occasions, most recently in the previous January, and always found to be negative. In fact she was the only person in the laboratory who did not have antibodies to EBV so her serum was highly prized as a negative control in the antibody test. However, when Diehl tested the blood sample he had taken during her illness in August it was highly positive. So Hutkin had seroconverted to EBV, either sometime before or during an attack of infectious mononucleosis. Furthermore, Diehl recalls that whereas in January her lymphocytes showed no signs of spontaneous transformation, now they 'grew in culture like crazy'. This rapid, outgrowth of cell lines from the blood of people with infectious mononucleosis was similar to that recently noted by Pope[40] and the findings from Hutkin's blood now gave a possible explanation.

All this pointed to the exciting possibility that infectious mononucleosis resulted from a primary EBV infection.[41] Fate, chance, luck, destiny—call it what you will—if Hutkin's serum had not been used as a negative control in the EBV antibody test, if Gertrude Henle had not insisted on her coming to the laboratory, if Hutkin had refused to come, or even delayed her visit for a week or so, the diagnosis and its overwhelming implications could have been missed.

Nevertheless, a single case of EBV seroconversion during an attack of acute infectious mononucleosis could just be coincidence. So now the race was on to check whether EBV was indeed the cause of the disease. The quickest way to get this proof was to find a doctor who had the relevant blood samples stored and ready to test. The Henles knew just who to call. James Niedermann ran the student health clinic at Yale University in New Haven, New England and had a longstanding interest in infectious mononucleosis. Fortunately, he was conducting an ongoing study on the disease at the time and had the ideal material ready and waiting—paired serum samples taken from students before and after an attack of infectious mononucleosis.

On testing these samples for EBV antibodies, the virus' association with the disease was confirmed. All those who developed infectious mononucleosis during the study (diagnosed by a positive heterophile antibody test) were EBV seronegative before the illness and seroconverted to become EBV antibody positive during the illness. Conversely, none of those who were EBV seropositive at entry to university subsequently developed infectious mononucleosis. Most of the acute cases had EBV antibody levels as high as those seen in Burkitt Lymphoma, and on recovery from the disease these levels declined but remained detectable long term. As the group reported in their landmark paper published in 1968: 'The evidence strongly implies that EB virus is etiologically related to infectious mononucleosis.[42]

Following this revelation, it was soon found that infectious EBV was present at high levels in the saliva of almost all infectious mononucleosis patients and at lower levels in at least 10 per cent of EBV carriers.[43] Thus, as Hoagland had deduced from case

53

histories, the virus is spread by salivary contact. The classic routes between family members are kissing and sharing of eating utensils, while among children the sharing of sucked toys is suggested as a likely method of transmission. Both these routes are likely to deliver a small dose of virus and generally result in a silent primary infection. On the other hand, kissing adolescents or young adults may transfer larger doses, and possibly this large dose is instrumental in inducing the symptoms of infectious mononucleosis.

* * *

In the Henles' research group, discussion now centred on the question of how infectious mononucleosis related to Burkitt Lymphoma. Were the two diseases both manifestations of primary EBV infection? Or did infectious mononucleosis precede Burkitt Lymphoma in African children? Did concurrent malaria infection perhaps drive infectious mononucleosis to become a malignant disease? In June 1968 Diehl headed for Kenya to find the answers. He worked with Peter Clifford at Kenyatta Hospital in Nairobi, collecting samples from hundreds of children living in East Africa and testing them for EBV antibodies. The results were unequivocal—wherever he looked, in the healthy and the sick, 85 to 95 per cent of adults had EBV antibodies. Even 45 per cent of children as young as 1 year had been infected with EBV and by 2 years of age this percentage had risen to adult levels. While searching unsuccessfully for cases of infectious mononucleosis in East Africa, Diehl met Denis Burkitt. He describes Burkitt as 'One of the most exciting figures I ever met—very humble, very pious, very strong minded and extremely opinionated'. On asking Burkitt if he had ever seen a case of infectious mononucleosis the great man laughed and replied, 'How would I know? Look at these people…they all have tonsillitis, they all have lymphadenopathy, they all have hepatosplenomegaly and they all have fever!'

In their report on the results from Africa, the Henle group compared the age of acquisition of EBV antibodies in East African populations with those in the US (Figure 9).[44] These differed markedly, with a much slower acquisition rate in the US, indicating that here EBV infection generally occurs later in life. Interestingly, they also reported that socioeconomic status made quite a difference to the age of infection in the US. While 50 per cent of 5-year-old children with low socioeconomic status were already EBV infected, in high socioeconomic groups just 20 per cent of 5-year-olds had EBV antibodies. These figures presumably reflect the different levels of hygiene in the groups and also explain why Diehl did not find cases of infectious mononucleosis in East Africa—because virtually everyone was infected with EBV as a young child—and for the same reason infectious mononucleosis was less common in low than in high socioeconomic groups in the US. However, the authors conclude that infection in early childhood is generally asymtomatic.

When the association between EBV and infectious mononucleosis was made public there followed a flurry of studies on both sides of the Atlantic. Large prospective studies were set up at the US Military

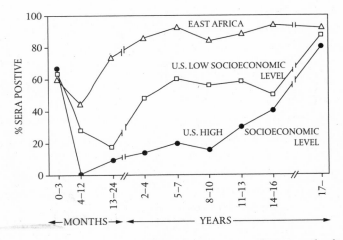

FIGURE 9 Chart showing the age of acquisition of EBV antibodies in East Africa and the US

Academy, West Point, New York, at Yale University, and at various universities and colleges in the UK to find out more about the virus and its spread in the target population for infectious mononucleosis.[45,46,47] The largest of these studies was at West Point, where approximately 1,400 cadets in the class entering in 1969 were enrolled in a four-year study. The participants were tested for past EBV infection at entry. Sixty-three per cent already had EBV antibodies while 37 per cent did not. Interestingly, only a few among the positive group recalled having suffered from infectious mononucleosis in the past, supporting the view that EBV infection in childhood is commonly silent. Also, among the EBV positive group, Afro-Caribbean cadets were over-represented (overall 81 per cent were EBV positive), as were those from the South Central States and those with a family income of under $6,000, while cadets from the more prosperous New England states were under-represented. These findings confirmed the previous study by the Henles and led the authors to speculate that the acquisition of EBV during childhood was influenced by socioeconomic status.

All the cadets were carefully monitored for illnesses suggestive of infectious mononucleosis throughout their four years at the academy, and the 437 cadets who were EBV negative at the start of the study were re-tested at the end of their four-year course. This revealed that 208 (46 per cent) had seroconverted. Of these, 53 (26 per cent) had developed classical heterophile antibody positive infectious mononucleosis. No cases of the disease occurred in cadets who were EBV antibody positive at entry to the study. From this and other studies scientists concluded that in Western societies:

- The majority of people experience primary EBV infection silently during childhood.
- The age distribution of EBV seropositivity in the US and Europe varies with socioeconomic status. Those in high socioeconomic groups are relatively protected from EBV infection during childhood.

- Only those who are EBV seronegative are susceptible to infectious mononucleosis.
- Among those acquiring EBV infection in adolescence or later, ~25 per cent develop the disease, the other ~75 per cent seroconvert silently.

In fact, in more recent studies tracking EBV seronegative students, those who reported the typical symptoms of infectious mononucleosis at the time of EBV seroconversion vary from 25 to 77 per cent.[48,49] In the study with the 77 per cent of overt disease, another 12 per cent of seroconverters developed non-classical, mild symptoms such as headache, body aches, and decreased appetite. Thus, in this study, 89 per cent had symptoms of some kind at the time of seroconversion, the severity of symptoms correlating directly with the level of virus in the blood. These variations suggest that primary EBV infection is usually symptomatic but that people differ in their threshold for reporting symptoms. For instance, college students may be more likely to consult a doctor for a headache, mild sore throat, or fever than would West Point cadets with a tough guy reputation to uphold.

**

After spending three and a half years in the Henles' laboratory, zur Hausen returned to Germany in 1969 to work at the Institute of Virology in Wurzburg. Here he put into practice the molecular techniques he had learnt in the US. He was able to demonstrate EBV DNA in all the cells in African Burkitt Lymphoma cell lines, even in those lines such as Raji which never produced virus particles.[50] This type of molecular evidence for the presence of the virus genome in a latent form in Burkitt Lymphoma cells was a major boost for the idea that EBV played a role in the development of the tumour, and later proved crucial in strengthening EBV's link to certain other types of cancer. Interestingly, despite the fact that he later made another major discovery—that human papilloma virus was the cause of cervical cancer—for which he is best known and was awarded a Nobel Prize in

2008, zur Hausen recalls that 'this work on EBV DNA detection was almost the best result I ever obtained because…it confirmed what I speculated from my student times—that human tumours contain the DNA of a latent virus'.

When Diehl left the Henles laboratory he went to work with a group of EBV researchers at the Karolinska Institute in Stockholm, Sweden, headed by another famous scientist, George Klein, who we meet again in the next chapter. Diehl then developed his own clinical research laboratory in Cologne, Germany, and became a leading expert on lymphoma, particularly Hodgkin Lymphoma.

After retirement from the diagnostic virology laboratory, the Henles continued with their research until shortly before Werner died in 1987 at the age of 76. Gertrude survived Werner by 19 years, dying in 2006. Their remarkable contribution identified EBV as a ubiquitous virus infection, as the cause of infectious mononucleosis, and as a transforming virus—major discoveries that greatly influenced how the EBV story developed over the following decades.

Still, by the end of the 1960s the question regarding the relationship between EBV and Burkitt Lymphoma remained unresolved. Was EBV a tumour virus or was it just a passenger virus in Burkitt Lymphoma cells? In the next chapter we will see how the largest field study ever carried out on African children, combined with some ingenious laboratory experiments, began to answer this all important question.

4

EBV in Africa:
Burkitt Lymphoma

Once several reports on Burkitt Lymphoma had been published the tumour began to cause quite a stir in the international scientific community. This may seem surprising considering that on a global scale its impact on child mortality was insignificant. At the time it caused just a few hundred deaths annually, and even within tropical Africa where it was the commonest childhood tumour it did not feature among the major childhood killers, of which gastroenteritis, pneumonia, and malaria topped the list. Nevertheless, scientists and doctors in several medical specialties were very excited by Burkitt's discovery, and felt that the tumour was of unique importance. Their view was that detailed study of Burkitt Lymphoma might provide vital clues to the cause and treatment of cancer in general, with implications far beyond the tumour itself.

First was its putative link to a virus—if this could be proved it would be the first example of a virus-associated tumour in humans—and possibly the first of many. Scientists argued that, even if only a small proportion of human cancers were caused by viruses, then, like smallpox and measles, the infection and therefore the disease might be preventable with vaccines.

Second, the tumour was supremely sensitive to chemotherapy, shrivelling away in days after a small dose of drugs. Twenty per cent of children with Burkitt Lymphoma were apparently cured by this approach at a time when the best that oncologists and radiothera-pists could offer for most other cancers was to halt their progression for a short while. They hoped to learn something from Burkitt Lymphoma's response to the drugs that would be applicable to other cancers.

Third, the clear geographic restriction of Burkitt Lymphoma, defined by temperature and rainfall, hinted at essential, environ-mental cofactors in addition to a virus that were required for the development of the tumour. Again, if these cofactors could be identified they might provide pointers to the cause of other, unre-lated cancers.

For all these reasons many local African doctors and scien-tists were now studying Burkitt Lymphoma, and several interna-tional teams of virologists, oncologists, and epidemiologists headed for equatorial Africa to do the same. For virologists the vital question was whether or not EBV really did cause Burkitt Lymphoma. This could only be answered by studies on the ground in Africa.

Accordingly, at the end of 1968, around 40 scientists gathered in 'one of Nairobi's less glamorous hotels for a round table conference on Burkitt Lymphoma'.[51] Their aim was to hammer out exactly what had to be done to find the answer. In addition to surgeons Burkitt and Clifford there were around 30 African doctors and scientists with firsthand experience of the tumour attending the meeting. The international experts included Gertrude and Werner Henle as well as George Klein from the Karolinska Institute in Stockholm. Also present was John Ziegler who the previous year had become the first director of the newly founded Uganda Cancer Institute in Kampala, and Gilbert Dalldorf, the distinguished American virologist now based in Nairobi. However, as things turned out the one person whose career would be most strongly influenced by this meeting was Guy de Thé, a medically trained tumour virologist from the International Agency for Research on Cancer in Lyon, France. Although he had not yet worked on EBV or Burkitt Lymphoma, he was destined to play a key role in implementing the bold, some thought over-ambitious, plans discussed at the meeting.

With the Henles' discovery of EBV as the cause of infectious mononucleosis fresh in everyone's mind, most of the delegates thought that Burkitt Lymphoma would similarly turn out to be directly linked to primary EBV infection. And, just like infectious mononucleosis, it must represent a rare outcome of the infection, because EBV is a common virus that usually infects silently. Perhaps again it was the result of a *delayed* primary infection. While it seemed that children in Africa were generally EBV infected by the age of 2, it was possible that this did not apply to every last one. Rare cases of delayed infection might mean a child first acquiring the virus at the age of 5 or 6, the very time that was the peak age for Burkitt Lymphoma development.

The ideal way to find out if this was the case was to mimic the classic studies such as the one on West Point cadets that showed conclusively that when cadets developed infectious mononucleosis, they also seroconverted to EBV (see chapter 3). This study had been completed in the four years that the cadets spent at the academy, but in the case of Burkitt Lymphoma the timescale might have to be much longer. The plan would be to collect blood samples from healthy young children living in a high-risk area for Burkitt Lymphoma in equatorial Africa. The samples would be stored while waiting for a few of the children to develop the tumour. The stored blood samples from these children, along with those from healthy control children, would then be tested for EBV antibodies to discover whether the Burkitt Lymphoma cases had been infected very recently or years earlier. The problem was that even in areas with the highest incidence of Burkitt Lymphoma the tumour affected less than one in a thousand children. So how many children must be studied to give a meaningful result? By the end of the meeting the number was agreed. Tens of thousands of young children would have to be enrolled in the study and provide a blood sample, in order to catch around 10 cases of the tumour developing within the following three years.

Theoretical plans for the study were set; however, most delegates went away convinced that this definitive experiment would never happen—it was too ambitious, too expensive, and politically too dangerous.[52] But de Thé had other ideas.

Guy de Thé (Figure 10) was born into the French aristocracy at a time when boys from such families were expected either to go into the church or the army. To the horror of his father, de Thé decided to become a doctor—the first ever in the de Thé dynasty. After spending several years studying avian tumour viruses at Duke University, North Carolina, US, in 1967 he was offered, and accepted, the post of head of the Human Tumour Virology Department at the new International Agency for Research on Cancer just opening in Lyon, France. This institute was funded by the World Health Organization (WHO) specifically to promote international collaborations in cancer research. The WHO was particularly keen to facilitate research in low-income countries through creating partnerships between international and local experts. Furthermore,

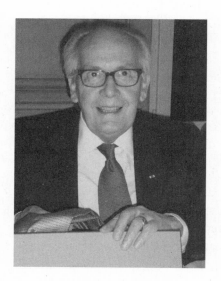

FIGURE 10 Guy de Thé

one of the stated aims of the agency was to identify the causes of cancer and implement preventative measures. To this end, the agency's mission statement declares that 'Emphasis is placed on elucidating the role of environmental and lifestyle risk factors and studying their interplay with genetic background in population-based studies....'[53] What could be more relevant than a study on Burkitt Lymphoma in Africa?

De Thé certainly regarded the proposed study as central to his remit at the Agency. On his return from Nairobi he lost no time in arranging a retreat in a remote location in the French Alps, where key members of the agency staff thrashed out the details and cost implications of such an enormously ambitious programme. Most important was to define a testable scientific hypothesis so that the study could be carefully planned to come up with the answer. In the end the complexity of the possible relationship between EBV and Burkitt Lymphoma meant that four separate hypotheses were proposed:[54]

1. That there was no causal relationship between EBV and Burkitt Lymphoma (the null hypothesis)
2. That the tumour develops shortly after primary EBV infection (the infectious mononucleosis model)
3. That the tumour develops in children who have an unusually long and heavy exposure to EBV
4. That EBV has a causal role in Burkitt Lymphoma but that a long time period between infection and tumour development allows for other factors to be involved (the cofactor hypothesis).

Several more meetings took place between interested parties to thrash out the details, but with some minor alterations the team eventually decided on a large prospective study modelled on the infectious mononucleosis studies and discussed at the meeting in Nairobi. In this scenario, differentiation between the various hypotheses depended entirely on variation in EBV antibody levels and patterns. If the null hypothesis (1 above) was correct, then EBV seroconversion would not be related to tumour development and there would be no difference in EBV antibody levels between children with Burkitt Lymphoma and control children. If the infectious mononucleosis model (2 above) was correct, then children who developed tumours would show signs of recent seroconversion to EBV at the time of tumour onset. If the tumour required a long and high exposure to EBV (3 above), then children with tumours would have seroconverted to EBV early in life and since then would have maintained higher levels of EBV antibodies than control children. The cofactor hypothesis (4 above), which could be viewed as an extension of model 3 with an additional interplay between EBV and other cofactors, could not be realistically pursued. To investigate this fully would require a research programme that was even larger, and last longer, than that planned, and this would be prohibitively more expensive.

Kuluva Hospital in the remote West Nile District of Uganda was chosen as the ideal base for the study. This was mainly because Ted Williams, a missionary doctor from the Kuluva hospital, had shown that the West Nile District had the highest incidence of Burkitt Lymphoma in Uganda. Williams had accompanied Burkitt on the long safari in 1961. He had been invited on the trip primarily because of his expertise in car maintenance, but his interest in Burkitt Lymphoma was obviously stimulated by what he saw. Having always kept detailed notes on all his patients, when he returned to Kuluva Hospital, Williams began to map the location of all the Burkitt Lymphoma cases he could trace in the region. Over a five-year period from 1961 to 1966 Williams identified over 50 known or suspected cases and produced some fascinating maps pinpointing the home villages of all the children he had seen suffering from the disease. In doing so he uncovered the highest incidence of the tumour in the whole of Uganda.

Williams took his maps to London to show to eminent epidemiologist Richard Doll, who discovered the link between smoking and lung cancer. Working alongside Doll at the MRC Statistics Unit in London was Malcolm Pike, who was looking into clustering of childhood leukaemia cases in the UK. He was very excited by Williams' maps and decided to go to Uganda to investigate further. Here he found tantalizing evidence of time–place clustering, meaning the tendency for several Burkitt Lymphoma cases to appear in the same location over a short period of time. This was unlike the random distribution of most other cancers, seeming more like an outbreak of an infectious disease and suggesting the involvement of a transmissible agent. Pike and Williams published these results in 1967[55] and from then on, despite its remote location, Kuluva Hospital became a centre for visiting researchers from around the world, all intent on studying Burkitt Lymphoma.

The few very rough roads and the virtual absence of transport in the area was a positive advantage to the study as it meant that the population (some 500,000 people from four separate tribes) remained very stable. Few people travelled far from their home village and so children enrolled in the study should be easy to trace year after year. The study area was to include the most densely populated regions in four adjacent counties—Aringa, Maracha, Terego, and Madi (Figure 11).

However, when de Thé asked WHO statistician, Nick Day, to look more carefully at the number of children needed in the study and the length of follow-up required to ensure a meaningful result, he came up with an enormous 40,000 newborns and babies followed up for 8 to 10 years. The cost was estimated at around one million US dollars per year, and de Thé recalls that when these figure were released he was strongly advised to abandon the study. But with the US National Cancer Institute willing to provide the cash through their Special Virus Cancer Program and through the Agency in Lyon, he was determined to carry on. So despite all the misgivings, the programme went ahead, jointly run by de Thé and Anton Geser, an epidemiologist from WHO.

Of course the logistics on the ground were horrendous. A small laboratory had to be built and equipped from scratch and the clinical facilities at Kuluva Hospital improved. Sixty staff were employed and trained as laboratory workers, drivers, phlebotomists, hospital

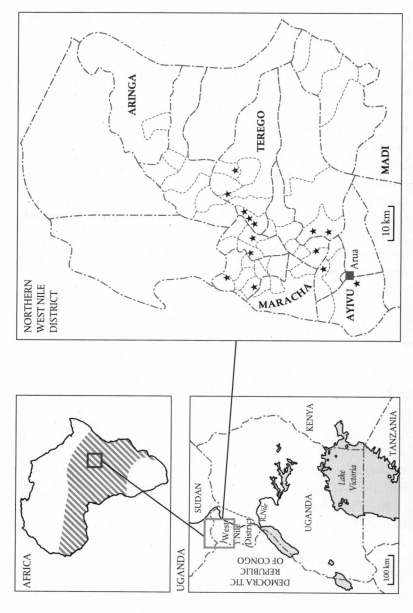

FIGURE 11 Maps showing the recruitment area for the EBV epidemiology study in West Nile District, Uganda

and health centre visitors, and case tracers. De Thé recalls that 'we were importing everything—4 or 5 Volkswagens, a Land Rover, tyres, gasoline, laboratory equipment, chemicals—it was just like a military operation.' The easiest way to get to Kuluva Hospital was to fly from Kampala to the capital of West Nile District, Arua, just eight miles from Kuluva. However, this would involve the expense of hiring a private plane and so was out of the question for the study. People and supplies all travelled the 300 miles north-west from Kampala to Arua by road, crossing the Albert Nile into the Northern Province at the new Pakwach Bridge. Peter Smith, an epidemiologist involved in the study, who lived at Kuluva for six months, recalls that it was a 12-hour trip on reasonably good roads. He generally camped in the Murchison Falls National Park overnight, and also liked to stop on Pakwach Bridge, which, he says, was an ideal place for photographing elephants.

Work on the project finally began in 1971, just as Idi Amin came to power in Uganda. When the full horror of Amin's dictatorship became known de Thé again came under pressure to quit. Fortunately though, the President was originally from the West Nile District and so was very supportive of the project, regarding it as 'his baby'. Nevertheless, the secret police were a threatening presence whose effects were unpredictable. On the one hand de Thé remembers that 'when we sent gasoline the secret police took half right away, so they liked us very much and we got a lot of things free'; on the other hand, Day says: 'Just as an organisational and human achievement, in Idi Amin's Uganda the success of the project was quite remarkable. As the country crumbled around them, the local staff kept it all on the road.'

Based in Lyon, de Thé and Geser held the purse strings and Geser visited Kuluva Hospital regularly every few months. De Thé made the occasional trip, each time insisting on travelling from Kampala to Arua accompanied by a high-ranking official from the Ministry of Health. Only then could he ensure safe passage over the Pakwach Bridge, where there was a checkpoint manned by trigger-happy soldiers with submachine guns. It was here that Smith recalls stopping for a bit of elephant spotting when a jeep full of gun-waving, Swahili-speaking soldiers materialized and demanded his camera. Without knowing a word of the language he somehow managed to negotiate keeping the camera for the loss of the film—with typical British understatement he describes the incident as 'a little bit unnerving'.

In order to recruit as many families as possible, the team held public meetings in each of the study areas to explain their plans. They then visited every household to register all its members. Locating all the remote households in the bush presented a problem but, as Day recalls: 'using aerial photographs of West Nile District taken in colonial times made a good starting point and then, in African style, one just went where the neighbours pointed'. Parents were asked to bring their children to a meeting point a few days later where they were enrolled in the study and had a small blood sample taken. Over 85 per cent of eligible children joined the study in Maracha, Terego, and Madi. However, recruitment was poor in Aringa, and so children in part of Ayivu County were also included (Figure 11).

Blood films were made from each sample to investigate malaria parasite load, then the serum was separated, frozen, and shipped in batches to the agency in Lyon for storage. Amazingly, by autumn 1972, the team had enrolled around 42,000 children aged between birth and 8 years old. This figure exceeded their target, and so in January 1973 the emphasis of the work changed from recruiting to searching for Burkitt Lymphoma cases. Children were visited around every six months in their villages and teams regularly called at all dispensaries, health centres, and hospitals in the study area, looking for likely Burkitt Lymphoma cases. When a suspected case was identified, Williams took biopsies of the tumour and these were sent for diagnosis to the Department of Pathology at Makerere University and to the Agency in Lyon where part of the biopsy was stored. The rest was coded and sent for evaluation to Burkitt Lymphoma specialists O'Conor, now at the US National Cancer Institute, and Wright, now at the University of Southampton, UK. Blood samples taken from children with Burkitt Lymphoma and members of their family were used for assessing the malaria parasite burden, and serum was stored for later measurement of antibodies to EBV and other viruses. Once this was accomplished, the affected children received the best of care. Around 40 per cent of them were still alive at the end of the study. De Thé attributes this high survival rate to early diagnosis resulting from heightened awareness among the study population and the intense surveillance by the local study team.

However, in November 1977 the EBV epidemiological study in Uganda was brought to a rather abrupt end. After around six years of funding, politicians, WHO officials, and leading scientists from the US Virus Cancer Programme began to question the enormous expense and the lack of results. Finally they withdrew the funding. By this time 31 children in the study area had developed Burkitt Lymphoma. But, disappointingly, only 14 of these had been enrolled at the beginning of the study and bled prior to tumour onset. The others were either not enrolled by their parents or were too old to be included in the original recruitment. Even so, this figure certainly represented fewer Burkitt Lymphoma cases than had been antici-pated among 42,000 children. Their stored serum samples were coded and analysed blind for EBV antibodies in three separate labo-ratories (in Lyon, Philadelphia, and Stockholm). Controls for each case included serum from a randomly chosen neighbouring child of the same age and sex taken at the time of diagnosis of the lymphoma, as well as sera from similarly matched children selected from the fro-zen bank of samples in Lyon.

The results were both surprising and remarkably clear-cut. All children who developed Burkitt Lymphoma had EBV antibodies long before the clinical onset of the tumour. This indicated that Burkitt Lymphoma was not, as had been suspected, the result of delayed primary EBV infection, and so its aetiology clearly differed from that of infectious mononucleosis. Moreover, all children with the tumour had a prior record of high levels of EBV antibodies when compared to controls. This could have indicated that the tumour arose in children with immune defects leading to overwhelming infections with persistent viruses like the herpes group viruses. However, the team excluded this possibility by testing for antibodies to other common herpesviruses (herpes simplex and cytomegalovirus). They found no significant differences in these antibody levels between cases and controls. Thus the increase was specific to EBV and suggested that the children carried an unusually heavy EBV infection for some years before the tumour developed. This result was decisive in distinguishing between the three hypotheses under test. In their publication in the journal *Nature* the team stated: 'These results strongly support our third hypothesis that children with long and heavy exposure to EBV are at increased risk of developing BL [Burkitt lymphoma].' This risk they estimated at around 30 times higher than that of age, sex, and locality matched controls. Finally they concluded: 'we therefore interpret our results as offering strong support for a causal relationship between EBV and BL [Burkitt lymphoma]'.[56]

Interestingly, with regard to malaria, they found no meaningful differences in the numbers of blood parasites between the Burkitt Lymphoma cases and controls. However, the authors continued to regard malaria as a possible factor involved in tumour development since it could so clearly account for the tumour's geographical restriction. At the end of the *Nature* report they mention the time–place clustering of Burkitt Lymphoma cases first documented by Williams and Pike. This was also noted, along with a seasonal variation of tumour incidence, in this new study. They suggested that this implied a short time interval (perhaps less than 18 months) between a final triggering event and the onset of Burkitt Lymphoma. Since primary EBV infection had undoubtedly occurred very early in life in these children, they proposed malaria infection in areas where malaria was holoendemic, meaning that it occurred all the year round, as this final trigger. Clearly this is a reasonable suggestion, but how might infection with a parasite predispose to a tumour?

It has long been known that recurrent attacks of malaria can cause both suppressed immunity and increased lymphocyte proliferation, the latter producing the grossly enlarged spleens often seen in patients with chronic malaria. More recently scientists have found that during an acute attack of malaria levels of EBV-infected lympho-cytes in the blood of African children rise quite dramatically, prob-ably due to a combination of both these effects. Since children living in holoendemic malaria areas are almost constantly infected with malaria parasites, at least until solid immunity is established at around 12 years of age, scientists argue that having increased num-bers of EBV-infected cells could predispose to Burkitt Lymphoma. However, both EBV and malaria are ubiquitous in tropical Africa, and yet Burkitt Lymphoma occurs in less than one in a thousand children. Clearly other factors, either genetic or environmental, must be required to realize the oncogenic potential of EBV.

* * *

While this huge epidemiological study was ongoing, some other breakthroughs in EBV research served to strengthen belief in a causative role for the virus in Burkitt Lymphoma. First, several researchers were attempting to satisfy Koch's postulate requiring that 'after being isolated and grown in culture the microbe can reproduce the disease in an experimental animal' (see chapter 2). Their aim was to mimic the clinical picture of both infectious mononucleosis and Burkitt Lymphoma in an animal model. As noted in chapter 3, small laboratory animals such as mice, rats, guinea pigs, and rabbits could not be infected by the virus, so researchers turned to using non-human primates. These species are generally large and expensive, and require special animal hous-ing facilities. Furthermore, today, experiments on primates are very strictly controlled by ethical considerations, not least the fact that many are endangered due to excessive hunting and/or loss of their forest habitats. However, this was not the case in the 1960s and 70s when they were often caught in the wild and sold specifi-cally for medical research.

Encouragingly, scientists found that when blood lymphocytes from several non-human primate species were infected with EBV in the laboratory they responded in the same way as human lym-phocytes—by transforming into permanently growing cell lines.

Despite this, many early attempts at infecting the animals themselves produced no evidence for infection or disease of any kind. We now realise that this was probably because primates often carry their own herpesviruses to which they develop antibodies. Some of these viruses are closely related to EBV so that the antibodies they generate recognize and inactivate EBV before it causes any disease. Indeed, when scientists tested blood from Old World (African and Asian) species such as chimpanzees, baboons, and African green, cynomologous, and rhesus monkeys, they often found antibodies that recognized EBV-producing cells in Burkitt Lymphoma cell lines. However not all animals of each species had these antibodies, and so the experiments continued using EBV seronegative animals. This showed that both chimpanzees and gibbons did seroconvert to become EBV antibody positive after infection with either EBV or with EBV-producing cell lines. So infections across the species barrier were possible. Thereafter, the challenge was to find the best dose of virus or cells to be given, the best route by which they were to be administered, and the most suitable choice of the animal species in which to look for evidence of virus-induced disease.

In late 1972 members of the Henles' research group in Philadelphia induced tonsillitis in two out of three gibbons (*Hylobates lar*) by injecting EBV directly into their tonsils.[57] All three animals seroconverted to EBV but all were negative for heterophile antibodies—the classical diagnostic test for infectious mononucleosis in patients. Despite not reproducing all aspects of the disease seen in humans, the work held out the hope that animal models would be informative in the future.

Yet no lymphomas developed in these gibbons so whether the virus was capable of causing cancer in experimental animals remained to be determined. However, in 1973 two more reports appeared from different laboratories, both with much more positive results. The two groups of scientists chose to infect New World (South American) primates because, in contrast to Old World primates, all such animals seemed to lack pre-existing antibodies that recognized EBV. In the first report to be published, Anthony Epstein and co-workers used owl monkeys (*Aotus trivirgatus*) in their experiments. These monkeys had been caught in the wild, either as immature or adult animals. Epstein injected EBV into three owl monkeys, keeping four other un-inoculated animals under identical conditions as controls. Only one of the inoculated animals became infected and this animal later developed a tumour and died after 14 weeks. At autopsy, enlarged, tumour-containing lymph glands were found all over the animal's body. The authors described this tumour as 'a striking reticuloproliferative disease very compatible with certain forms of malignant lymphoma'.[58] The tumour cells did not contain virus particles. However, Epstein later grew a cell line from one of the affected lymph glands and showed that, just like Burkitt Lymphoma cell lines, some cells in this line contained virus particles.

The second report came from George Miller and colleagues at Yale University, US, and used cottontop marmosets (*Saguinus Oedipus*, later called cottontop tamarins);[59] tiny, squirrel-sized primates that live in the forests of Columbia. A group of four animals were given EBV while four others acted as controls. Two animals from each group also received immune-suppressing drugs to see if this would increase the chances of EBV-related tumour formation. Three of the four EBV-inoculated animals, including both of those on immune suppression, developed tumours within 46 days, whereas all four control animals remained healthy throughout the experiment. Autopsies on the three tumour-bearing animals revealed widespread disease involving abdominal lymph glands, liver, lung, and intestine. Microscopic examination of the tumours showed that, regardless of anatomical site, all were lymphomas.

The results of these two animal studies proved that EBV was indeed an oncogenic virus, that is, it could cause cancer, at least when transmitted experimentally into certain New World primate species. The findings went a long way towards satisfying Koch's postulate for a causal link between EBV and Burkitt Lymphoma since the animal tumours were indeed lymphomas. However, it later became clear that they were distinct from the classic Burkitt Lymphoma in a number of respects (see chapter 6). Following Miller and colleagues' report, cottontop tamarins became the animal model of choice for studies on the mechanisms of EBV tumour development and prevention. As these animals bred well in captivity, were easy to handle because of their small size and regularly developed lymphomas after inoculation of EBV cottontop tamarins played a vital role in later work towards a vaccine.

* * *

Another key breakthrough in defining EBV infection as an essential element in the causation of African Burkitt Lymphoma came from the laboratory of George Klein and his wife, Eva, at the Karolinska Institute in Stockholm, Sweden (Figure 12). The Kleins both grew up in Budapest, Hungary, where they were school students at the time of the Nazi occupation. As Jews they were lucky to survive. In a moving account of their early struggles George writes: 'on the 10th of January 1945…I emerged from a cellar on the outskirts of Budapest where I had been hiding, with false papers, during the last weeks of

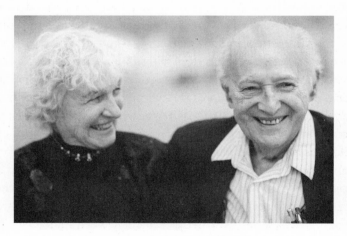

FIGURE 12　Eva and George Klein

the German occupation…I had survived in spite of an 80 per cent chance that I would end my 19 years in the gas chambers or military slave labor camps.'[60] It seems that a combination of chance and determination played a large part in the stories of the Kleins' early lives and work.

Both George and Eva were determined to study medicine. During the Nazi occupation this was not possible for those of Jewish descent, and in the following chaos of post-war, Russian-occupied Hungary it was certainly very difficult. In 1945 the university in Budapest was closed and so until it reopened George and Eva, unknown to each other at the time, both attended classes at the University of Szeged over 160 km away. They met by chance in 1947 while on holiday. But very soon George was offered the chance to travel to Stockholm with a group of students visiting Jewish Student Clubs in Sweden. As they said goodbye both thought they would never see each other again. This trip gave George the break he was looking for: while in Stockholm he procured a junior research assistant post at the Karolinska Institute. He only returned to Budapest briefly a few months later to marry Eva, and fortunately she managed to join him in Sweden in 1948, finding a way through the 'Iron Curtain' that now divided Europe into East and West. They have lived in Stockholm and worked together at the Karolinska Institute ever since.

For many years the Kleins studied the immune response generated by virus-induced lymphomas in mice, building one of the leading laboratories for tumour immunology. Then in the 1960s they decided to apply the experience they had gained from the mouse model to a human tumour, in particular a putative, virus-related tumour. The obvious choice was Burkitt Lymphoma. They contacted Peter Clifford, ENT surgeon at the Kenyatta Hospital in Nairobi, to request material, and thus began a long and fruitful collaboration. Clifford, who treated children with Burkitt Lymphoma every day, was particularly interested in whether the tumour's rapid response to chemotherapy was immune mediated, so he was happy to provide biopsy material for their experiments.

The Kleins are full of praise for Clifford. As the only ENT surgeon in East Africa at the time he was an extremely busy man but he always found the time to send them regular Burkitt Lymphoma biopsy samples. George recalls that 'the material...arrived with chronometric precision...Every Tuesday night was "Burkitt night"...It was not difficult to motivate our personnel to work through the night every Tuesday.'[61]

Soon after beginning this work the Kleins found antibodies in the blood of Burkitt Lymphoma patients that reacted with cells in Burkitt Lymphoma cell lines. These antibodies detected a virus protein expressed on the outer membrane of a proportion of Burkitt Lymphoma cells, and so the Kleins called it 'membrane antigen'. Unlike the antibodies picked up by the Henles' fluorescent viral capsid antigen test described in chapter 2, which only reacted with the few virus-producing cells, these antibodies reacted with around 10 per cent of cells in Burkitt Lymphoma cell lines. This was the first hint that EBV was present in more cells than just those that produced virus particles. But it still did not exclude the possibility that EBV was just a passenger virus coincidentally carried by Burkitt Lymphoma cell cultures and not present in every cell. Interestingly, measuring antibodies against membrane antigen had some prognostic significance for Burkitt Lymphoma patients. Levels were usually high at diagnosis and tended to remain high in those patients who responded well to chemotherapy. However, they fell if chemotherapy failed to control the tumour. Moreover, a drop in their level in long-term survivors often heralded a tumour relapse.

In 1970 the Kleins teamed up with Harald Zur Hausen, now back in Germany at the Institute of Virology in Wurzburg, who had by this time developed a molecular probe that could detect EBV DNA inside latently infected cells. Using this on Burkitt Lymphoma specimens, they demonstrated the presence of multiple copies of EBV DNA in all the malignant cells of at least 97 per cent of African Burkitt Lymphomas, and in cell lines derived from them. Importantly, this held true even for the African Burkitt Lymphoma cell lines such as

Raji that never made virus particles (see chapter 3).[62] This finding consolidated the link between EBV and African Burkitt Lymphoma but, ironically, the same approach showed that only 10 to 15 per cent of sporadic Burkitt Lymphoma occurring in children in the West were positive for the virus. It seemed that the link between virus and tumour was strong but only with respect to the high incidence, endemic form of the disease.

Focusing on African tumours scientists at the Karolinska Institute began to ask how EBV was maintained, even in cell lines like Raji. Surprisingly, they showed that each cell carried multiple copies of the virus genome in the form of miniature circles of DNA that were present in the cell nucleus alongside, but separate from, the cell's own chromosomes. This insight immediately explained how EBV infection is maintained in cells. The virus makes its genome into a mini-chromosome, so that as the cell duplicates its own DNA in preparation for dividing into two daughter cells, the virus genome is also faithfully duplicated and passed on to those new cells in just the same way.[63]

This was certainly a step forward, but critics then asked the question: how can a latent virus inside a cell induce those cells to proliferate and cause a tumour? It seemed reasonable to expect that at least some viral proteins must be made in the malignant cells. The race was on to find an EBV-encoded protein present in every cell in EBV-related Burkitt Lymphoma. Early work from John Pope's laboratory in Australia had suggested that African Burkitt cell lines, even the Raji cell line that lacked virus-producing cells, contained a 'soluble antigen' that seemed to be a marker of EBV infection.[64] But if this antigen was important in linking EBV infection to tumour growth, it would need to be present in every single cell.

The breakthrough came in 1973 when a junior member of John Pope's research group in Australia, Beverly Reedman, spent a year as a visiting research fellow in the Kleins' laboratory. On arrival at the Karolinska Institute Reedman recalls that: 'I was warmly welcomed, although everyone asked where I would be working as there was so little space ... an immediate sign of a highly productive lab.' Describing her work she continues: 'I began dabbling with conventional immunofluorescence staining of Burkitt Lymphoma cell lines. Using the strongest EBV-reactive sera, I detected some faint staining in a large proportion of the cells...so George [Klein] suggested trying to enhance this with a third step in the immunofluorescence "sandwich". The result was amazing. I saw beautiful nuclear staining in virtually every cell...not just in all EBV positive cell lines...but also in freshly prepared Burkitt Lymphoma cells from the Tuesday night delivery from Nairobi.'

Reedman and Klein called this antigen EBNA, for **EB**V-encoded **n**uclear **a**ntigen. This was a hugely important discovery at the time, providing the first clear evidence that the viral genome was not just present but also active in every Burkitt tumour cell. This was a crucial step in identifying EBV as a key factor in the causation of the tumour. For the next 10 years EBNA, as defined by the immunoflourescence staining technique, was to remain the only detectable marker of the virus' active presence either in tumours or in cell lines.

Much later, as knowledge of the virus increased and new detection systems were developed, five other EBNAs were discovered. As a result Reedman and Klein's EBNA was re-christened 'EBNA1'. Nevertheless, EBNA1 remains the first, and arguably the most important, of the six EBNAs, because it is still the only viral protein that is made in Burkitt Lymphoma cells.[65]

* * *

By the mid 1970s it seemed that most of the pieces of the Burkitt Lymphoma/EBV puzzle had fallen into place. But still one issue remained unresolved—what was the rare genetic or environmental cofactor that was postulated to co-operate with EBV and malaria to cause the tumour? Ironically, that third cofactor turned out to be the most crucial of all, one that was involved, not just in the EBV-associated African form of the tumour, but in all cases of Burkitt Lymphoma worldwide. It was even present in all those rare cases seen in Western countries where there was no malaria, and where only a minority of the tumours were EBV DNA-positive. This third cofactor came from a genetic accident, occurring by chance in the chromosomes of a rare cell destined to give rise to the tumour and driving the tumour's very rapid growth. Genetic accidents of one form or another underpin the development of almost all forms of cancer, but in many cases their effects on the genome of cancer cells are quite subtle and often only detectable by DNA sequencing. Only in a few types of cancers are these accidents visible at the level of gross chromosome structure but, fortunately, one such cancer turned out to be Burkitt Lymphoma. The first clue came from George and Yanka Manolov, a Bulgarian husband and wife team who were working in George Klein's laboratory at the time.

When the Manolovs arrived at the Karolinska Institute, a new staining technique had just been developed that could reveal specific banding patterns on human chromosomes, allowing changes in their overall structure to be described more accurately than before. George Klein suggested that the Manolovs use this new technique to study the chromosomes in Burkitt Lymphoma cells. Accordingly, they stained up the chromosomes in cells from biopsies sent by Clifford and, to everyone's surprise, found a consistent abnormality. In the tumour cells there was an extra band attached to one of the chromosome 14 pair that was not present in the chromosomes of normal cells from the same patients. The discovery of a chromosome change that was specific to the Burkitt tumour aroused much interest when the work was published in 1972,[66] but it was another decade before its true significance was fully appreciated.

When the Manolovs returned to Bulgaria George Klein turned to the Karolinska's resident chromosome expert, Lore Zech, to continue the study. In addition to the extra band on one chromosome 14, she noticed that one of the chromosome 8 pair was abnormally short in Burkitt Lymphoma cells. In fact she had discovered an 8:14 translocation, meaning that a piece of chromosome 8 had accidentally broken off and attached to the end of chromosome 14.[67] The great majority of Burkitt tumours had this common 8:14 translocation, always involving attachment between the same regions of those two chromosomes. However, a few cases showed different patterns, involving an attachment between chromosome 8 and a particular part of either chromosome 2 or 22; these were the so-called variant translocations 2:8 and 8:22. Interestingly, the same region of chromosome 8 seemed to be involved in all three cases, an observation that was later to become hugely significant. More important at the time was the fact that, in any individual tumour, every cell carried the same translocation.

Tumours generally arise from a single rogue progenitor cell and so, in the case of Burkitt Lymphoma, the translocation must have been present in that progenitor cell before it became fully malignant and began to grow. Such a finding greatly strengthened the argument that the translocation was not a secondary change occurring in just some of the tumour cells as a consequence of uncontrolled growth, but was a crucial step in the sequence of events that had actually caused the tumour. Burkitt Lymphoma was one of the first human tumours to be linked with a specific set of chromosome translocations. The effect was to give this rare African lymphoma an even greater starring role as one of the most fascinating of human malignancies.

But as with all important findings, this raised yet more questions. While the Burkitt Lymphoma-associated chromosome translocations were almost certainly a critical factor in the tumour's development, what were their effects in molecular terms? Exactly how did such translocations contribute to malignant change? It took a momentous breakthrough by two American scientists, Michael Bishop and Harold Varmus, working on a completely different virus-associated cancer, the now famous Rous sarcoma, to provide the vital clue. Their work, first published in 1976 and recognized by award of the Nobel Prize for Physiology or Medicine in 1989, proved the existence of oncogenes. These are normal cellular genes that, if mutated and/or released from their normal controls, can serve as one step in the conversion of normal cells into cancer.

How did these revelations relate to the chromosome translocations seen in Burkitt Lymphoma? The answer came when the genes involved in the three sets of translocations, 8:14, 2:8, and 8:22, were identified. It turned out that the three chromosomes that were partners for chromosome 8 in the different types of translocation, chromosomes, 14, 2, and 22, had something very interesting in common. They were the three chromosomes that contained the immunoglobulin genes that code for antibody (or immunoglobulin) molecules. These genes are specifically active in antibody-producing B lymphocytes, the cell type from which Burkitt Lymphoma arose. What's more, the translocations seen in Burkitt Lymphoma broke chromosome 14, 2, or 22 at exactly the point where those immunoglobulin genes lay. Even more importantly, the breakpoint on chromosome 8 in each case turned out to be near one of the best-known cellular oncogenes called c-myc. In each case, therefore, the translocation had moved the c-myc oncogene from its normal location and placed it next to an active immunoglobulin gene. The result was to release the oncogene from its usual tight controls and allow it to be highly active. This led to unusually high levels of the c-myc protein being made, a protein that delivers a very powerful growth signal to the affected cell.

The fact that Burkitt Lymphoma can occur as a rare disease in the West without the involvement of either EBV or malaria as a cofactor clearly shows that the translocation itself carries a risk of the affected cell acquiring further accidental genetic changes and moving on to become fully malignant. But that risk is low. By contrast, the path to malignancy seems to be greatly accelerated in the presence of sustained high-level EBV infection and chronic malaria, cofactors that underpin the high incidence, African form of the disease. So how could these two cofactors work?

The first clue comes from careful analysis of the chromosomal translocations at the molecular level. This strongly suggests that they have arisen as accidents of a particular phase of the B lymphocyte's life history when it is busy mounting an active antibody response. It turns out that one of the side effects of chronic malarial infection is that it stimulates B lymphocytes, inducing antibody responses that are unusually large, yet unable to neutralize the parasite. This chronic stimulation of B lymphocyes and activation of antibody production must greatly increase the chance of an accidental 8:14, 2:8, or 8:22 translocation happening, thereby creating a larger pool of cells on the brink of conversion to malignancy. Now we can add EBV into the picture. This virus naturally establishes a latent infection in B lymphocytes and it is normally carried by around one in a million of these cells in the blood of healthy, EBV seropositive people in the West. The stimulatory effect of malaria greatly increases the number of EBV-positive B lymphocytes in the blood, so that children in tropical Africa often have levels 100 to 1000-fold higher than those seen in the West. This sounds dramatic, but still less than 1 per cent of an African child's B lymphocytes carry the virus. Therefore the random chance of any B lymphocyte tumour being EBV-positive is also less than 1 per cent. Yet almost every case of African Burkitt Lymphoma has arisen from an EBV-infected cell. This strongly suggests that the virus somehow increases the chances of a myc gene translocation-positive cell achieving full malignancy. How could that be?

That question puzzled researchers for many years, until the first hints of a solution came from scientists at Hokkaido University in Japan. In 1994, they had been studying a cell line established from a rare EBV-positive case of Burkitt Lymphoma in a Japanese child. The cell line was very unusual because in culture some of the growing cells lost the virus genome and became EBV DNA-negative. For the first time, it was possible to compare the behaviour of EBV-positive and EBV-negative cells, all derived from the same tumour. Clearly the cells could grow equally well under favourable conditions, whether or not they contained the virus. However, when deprived of nutrients or placed under unfavourable culture conditions, the EBV-positive cells survived better than the cells that had lost the virus genome.[68] It later turned out that the EBV-loss cells were dying by a process known as 'apoptosis'. This is a kind of cellular suicide which, during normal development, all B lymphocytes are programmed to commit if they are no longer deemed to be useful to the immune system. So, even though Burkitt Lymphoma cells are malignant, they still carry an innate sensitivity to apoptosis that reflects their origin as B lymphocytes. Anything that reduces the apoptosis sensitivity of pre-malignant B lymphocyte cells will increase their chance of growing out successfully as a tumour.

Ironically, therefore, even though EBV can transform normal B lymphocytes into permanently growing cell lines in the laboratory, the virus' contribution to the development of Burkitt Lymphoma is not growth transformation. Growth is driven by the uncontrolled c-myc oncogene. Instead, EBV's role in this particular context is to provide a survival advantage to the c-myc-expressing cell. How the virus does this is still not fully understood, in fact it is an important area of present-day research. As ever, there are more questions to answer. But for the moment, let us bring the story of EBV and Burkitt Lymphoma to a conclusion. While in rare cases the tumour can arise without the involvement of EBV, on a global scale the great majority of Burkitt cases are EBV genome-positive and, in such cases, the virus is almost certainly important in producing the tumour. In effect, we are as close as we can be to fulfilling Koch's postulates with respect to EBV and Burkitt Lymphoma. So far, so good, but the Burkitt tumour is just one part of a much bigger picture as far as EBV's associations with human cancer are concerned. To see how that picture began to unfold we have to go back to the virus' discovery and to another set of surprise findings.

5

EBV in Asia:
Nasopharyngeal carcinoma

The mid-1960s saw the newly-born field of EBV research in a state of flux. It was the Burkitt tumour's highly unusual geographic distribution that had first caught Anthony Epstein's attention, prompting the hunt for a virus that was restricted to equatorial regions of Africa. Yet the virus found in Burkitt Lymphoma cells, far from being geographically restricted, appeared to be carried as a harmless infection by most people on the planet. What's more, although EBV was found in association with African Burkitt Lymphoma, the same tumour occurred sporadically in the West where most cases did not contain the virus. As happens so often in science, the sense of excitement that comes with any new discovery begins to pale as the floodgates open and more information, often contradictory, pours in. The notion that EBV was an oncogenic agent seemed premature in the extreme.

It was in just these circumstances that the story took a new and completely unexpected turn which, in time, was to greatly strengthen the virus's links to malignant disease. It began with a chance finding that arose from the study of Burkitt Lymphoma in Africa, but from there led to a quite different tumour, also with a marked geographic distribution, this time with an epicentre in South East Asia. By 1966, the discovery of EBV two years earlier had caught the attention of many cancer researchers around the world. One of these was Lloyd

Old, a leading immunologist at the Memorial Sloan-Kettering Institute in New York. Old's main interest was in the immune response to cancers induced by RNA viruses in mice. However, when his colleague Herbert Oettgen returned to New York after working with Peter Clifford in Nairobi, he persuaded Old to look at anti-tumour immune responses in Burkitt Lymphoma patients. Using a standard method that detected antigen–antibody interactions he tested African sera provided by Clifford for reactivity against a crude antigen preparation made from an EBV-producing Burkitt Lymphoma cell line. The method was relatively insensitive, and so only sera with high antibody levels gave a positive reaction. Sure enough, sera from African Burkitt Lymphoma patients were much more frequently positive than were sera from healthy control donors or from the few patients they tested with other types of leukaemia or lymphoma. However, among the control samples, Clifford had included sera from patients with a tumour called 'carcinoma of the post-nasal space' which, as an ENT surgeon, he saw quite frequently in his Nairobi clinic. Surprisingly, an even higher proportion of these patients' sera tested positive than did the African Burkitt Lymphoma sera.[69]

The finding was not just unexpected but also unwelcome. This was their first attempt to include patients with other types of cancer as controls in the antibody screening assays and it had already detected another tumour with high EBV antibody levels. To most observers, this weakened the argument that EBV's association with Burkitt Lymphoma was specific. The only way to maintain the significance of that association was to suggest that the virus was also linked to this second tumour type. But it was hard to believe that, by chance, the investigators had stumbled upon a second EBV-associated tumour. Indeed there were serious scientific objections to the virus being linked with a cancer of this particular type. At that time, all the available evidence suggested that EBV only infected lymphocytes, yet cancer of the post-nasal space was a tumour of epithelial cells, the cells that line body surfaces.

While carcinoma of the post-nasal space was rare in the Western world, surveys showed that a specific form of this tumour, where the epithelial cells had a distinct undifferentiated appearance, was more frequent in some parts of North and East Africa, and was especially common throughout the populous regions of South East Asia. This was particularly the case in Southern China where the disease was, and still is, one of the most common tumours in men, with incidence rates as high as 20 to 30 per 100,000 people per year, and second only to cervical cancer in women. The possibility of a link between EBV and carcinoma of the post-nasal space seemed bizarre, but it could not be completely discounted. After all, the EBV story owed its very existence to Burkitt Lymphoma, a disease previously unknown to the Western world, so why not another unusual tumour? As interest grew, the post-nasal space tumour was re-christened 'nasopharyngeal carcinoma', a name that was more anatomically correct but still did not roll easily off the tongue, hence the abbreviation to its acronym 'NPC'.

The first thing to resolve was whether the findings of Old and colleagues, measuring antibodies against a crude mixture of antigens from a Burkitt Lymphoma cell line, could be reproduced using the immunofluorescence assays being developed by Gertrude and Werner Henle and George Klein (see chapters 3 and 4). These assays detected antibodies against three defined sets of EBV proteins present in virus-producing cells, the virus capsid and membrane antigens described earlier, and another complex called early antigen. Futhermore, these assays were much more sensitive and could accurately determine the levels of those antibodies by testing sera at several different dilutions. Knowing the antibody level was critical because most healthy, EBV-infected people were positive for capsid, membrane and, in some cases, also early antibodies. So the question was whether these antibody responses were unusually strong in NPC patients. It did not take long to show that this was indeed the case. Patients with NPC had much higher EBV antibody levels than healthy people or indeed patients with other types of head and neck cancer, whereas their antibody responses to other common viruses were in the normal range. Against all odds, there really did seem to be a special connection between EBV and NPC.

These findings, based on patients with the tumour in East Africa, immediately caught the attention of John Ho, a clinician who dealt with large numbers of NPC patients in his daily practice in Hong Kong. Ho, widely known as 'The Emperor' in his native city, was a remarkable leader and had long been a pioneer of research into the carcinoma that he called the 'Cantonese tumour'. Now the link with EBV gave that research new impetus. Assays on sera from his patients quickly showed that NPC in China was likewise associated with high EBV antibody levels. So the connection between virus and tumour extended right into the heartland of high NPC incidence, in South East Asia. What's more, the Hong Kong studies also showed that EBV antibody levels seemed to correlate with the disease course, such that patients progressing to later stage disease showed increasing levels, while the levels often fell following successful treatment.

Consequently, by 1970, the possibility of a causal link between EBV and NPC was gaining credibility, but the evidence was based entirely on increased antibody responses. This alone was not enough. We have seen how it took detection firstly of the EBV genome, secondly the virus coded nuclear antigen, EBNA, before many were convinced of the significance of EBV's association with Burkitt Lymphoma. Similarly, in the early 1970s the application of these techniques to NPC was paramount. Could the epithelial cells of NPC really be EBV-infected or was there another explanation for the tumour's apparent relationship to EBV? A different explanation seemed eminently possible because NPC tissue contained large numbers of non-malignant lymphocytes alongside the epithelial tumour cells. Indeed this picture was so typical of NPC that many textbooks at the time referred to the tumour as a 'lymphoepithelioma'. If these non-malignant lymphocytes were EBV-infected, rather than the malignant epithelial cells, then that could explain why NPC patients made strong antibody responses to the virus. Faced with this dilemma, the race was on to find out whether EBV DNA could be detected in NPC tumour tissue and, if so, which cell type carried the virus.

Both Harald zur Hausen in Germany and other scientists in the US began applying their molecular methods of detecting the virus genome to NPC and found that EBV DNA was indeed present, often at levels which approached those seen in African Burkitt Lymphoma.[70,71] Crucially, zur Hausen then adapted these methods to detect EBV DNA within individual cells, a technique called 'in situ hybridization', and found that the virus was actually present in the malignant epithelial cells.[72] Furthermore, in Sweden, Klein and colleagues, using the EBNA immunofluorescence test developed in their laboratory the previous year, showed that these same epithelial cells were EBNA-positive.[73] So by 1974 it was clear that EBV's association with NPC was every bit as significant as it was with Burkitt Lymphoma. Moreover, the EBV/NPC connection seemed even firmer because it transcended the barriers of geography and disease incidence. Whereas the virus was consistently present only in Burkitt Lymphoma in its high incidence form in equatorial Africa and New Guinea, EBV was present in all cases of undifferentiated NPC, whether occurring at high incidence in South East Asia, at intermediate incidence in certain areas of Africa, or at low incidence in the West.

These molecular studies generated much interest and brought NPC into the scientific spotlight. By contrast, a short report appearing in the medical literature the following year seemed much more mundane, yet in its own way, was destined to be just as influential. Its authors, Arthur Ammann and his colleagues in San Francisco, were not specifically interested in NPC but were studying a question of general interest in cancer research at that time: whether radiation treatment for cancer might have secondary effects on the patient's immune system. As Ammann recalls: 'My research fellow's husband was working in the radiation oncology department. We frequently had joint discussions and I asked him if we could look at some of his patients who were having radiation treatment. Of course we could have selected other cancers but, as it happened, he was treating a number of patients with nasopharyngeal carcinoma from the large Chinese community in San Francisco.' Part of that study was to measure these patients' ability to respond to common vaccines. While doing so, the researchers happened to notice that total levels of one class of serum antibodies, the IgA antibodies, were consistently between two- and five-fold higher than usual in individuals with NPC, whereas levels of the more common IgG and IgM antibody classes were normal.[74] The reason for this was completely unclear but, the authors asked, if increased IgA levels were really specific to this type of tumour, could this have something to do with the tumour's resident virus, EBV?

As with so many important advances in the early years of EBV research, it was the Henles who provided the answer. All their early studies showing elevated EBV antibodies in NPC patients had focused on the conventional IgG response. Now they adapted their immunofluorescence assays to specifically detect IgA antibodies. Within a year they had completed the key experiments. The results were remarkable.[75] Almost all NPC patients had detectable IgA responses to the EBV capsid antigen and many also to early antigen, whereas such antibodies were rarely seen in healthy controls or in patients with other head and neck tumours. So IgA responses to the virus were a highly specific marker of individuals with NPC. Once again, within individual patients, the level of these antibodies correlated with tumour burden, increasing with disease progression and gradually decreasing after successful treatment. So IgA antibodies to EBV were potentially useful both as a diagnostic tool to identify patients with NPC and as a means of tracking how a patient responded to therapy. This idea of a simple blood test for NPC had particular resonance for Southern Chinese populations, especially in the highest affected regions of Gaungzhou and Guangxi where

NPC was a major public health concern. In these areas, not only did the disease occur at high incidence but also, unlike most tumours which tend to strike in old age, it preferentially affected people, especially men, in their forties or fifties, at a time when they were still in the prime of their working life.

When the Henles' IgA antibody findings were published in 1976, they made a huge impression on a microbiologist working at the Central Health Institute in Beijing. The microbiologist's name was Zeng Yi, a charismatic figure who proudly traces his family dynasty back through 76 generations to the famous Chinese philosopher Zeng Zi, disciple of Confucius. The modern-day Zeng had been born in Southern China, had studied medicine at the epicentre of NPC incidence in Guangzhou, and knew all about the ravages of this tumour. He immediately decided to explore the possibility of using the IgA antibody response to EBV as a means of detecting early-stage disease. Zeng and his team did not believe in doing things by halves. Inspired by the massive prospective study that Guy de Thé and colleagues had just completed in Uganda (see chapter 4), the indomitable Zeng aimed at a study group that would eventually rise to more than four times the Ugandan cohort. Not for nothing did he become known as 'Guy de Thé's twin brother'!

Their study site was the city of Wuzhou and the surrounding area of Zangwu County, in the centre of the high NPC incidence region of Guangxi. Between 1978 and 1980, blood samples were taken from many thousands of adults, the sera frozen, and then air-freighted to Beijing for antibody screening. When asked about the difficulties he encountered with such a massive study, Zeng replied with characteristic good humour: 'Well, some people would not allow us to collect their blood. Once a middle-aged woman said to us "if you try to collect my blood I'll jump into the river". She really did jump...luckily the river was not deep and we rescued her immediately...Finally she agreed to give a few drops of blood for the survey.' Not surprisingly, these kinds of anecdotes do not make it into scientific reports, but they give a flavour of the logistic problems with which such large population surveys had to contend, albeit in an age that pre-dated today's much stricter rules over participants' consent.

The results were described in two landmark reports, published in 1982 and 1983 respectively.[76,77] The first study enrolled almost 13,000 people living in Wuzhou city who were 40 to 59 years old, the peak age for NPC development. While essentially all were EBV-infected and therefore positive for IgG antibodies to the virus, only 30 individuals had IgA responses to both the capsid and early antigens and, of these, a staggering 30 per cent (9/30) had hitherto unrecognized NPC. Boosted by this massive screening exercise, the number of new NPC cases diagnosed per year in Wuzhou city was twice the average annual number seen in the 1970s, with a marked skewing towards patients with early stage, and therefore more treatable, disease. This led to an even larger study, albeit focusing only on the capsid antibody response, but involving nearly 150,000 subjects aged 30 or above from the whole of Zangwu county, including Wuzhou. This identified 3,500 individuals with IgA capsid antibodies, of whom 55 already had hitherto-unrecognized NPC, and a further 32 developed the disease over the following three years. This clearly showed that, in Chinese people, the presence of IgA antibodies to the virus pinpointed a small fraction of the population who were at particularly high risk of NPC and could be monitored regularly for signs of early disease. Screening of this kind still goes on in high NPC incidence areas of Southern China to this day,[78] a testament to the impact of these first pioneering studies.

* * *

If EBV is a necessary link in the long chain of events leading to NPC, then it raises many questions. Here is a virus that is present in all human populations yet is linked to a cancer that shows such remarkable variation in incidence in different parts of the world. Could the geography of disease incidence reflect genetic differences between populations in their susceptibility to NPC, or differences in exposure to a second environmental co-factor, or both? Exploring these questions will take us away from the EBV story for a little while, but will bring us back better equipped to understand what the virus is doing in this fascinating tumour.

A good place to start the exploration is with some simple but telling observations on NPC incidence among the world-wide diaspora of Cantonese-speaking people. Over centuries, Cantonese people migrated throughout South East Asia, and in many places, for example in Indonesia, they gradually integrated into the population through several generations of inter-marriage with indigenous people. In these circumstances, their Chinese ethnicity becomes diluted. By contrast, more recent migrations to far-flung destinations generated younger communities which maintained their Chinese ethnicity over at least three generations. The best example is on the US West Coast where the California Gold Rush began the first wave of migration around 1850 and where even the US Government's Chinese Exclusion Act of 1882 did not prevent the establishment of thriving Chinese communities. As a result, epidemiologists were able to look at disease incidence in significantly large numbers of such people, comparing first generation migrants (born in China) to their locally born children and grandchildren.

The results of studies carried out in the US in the 1970s showed a trend which has since been confirmed, not just within the US but for other Chinese migrations outside of Asia. The incidence of NPC among first generation migrants was as high as that in their Cantonese homeland even though their tumours typically developed many years after they had left China. By contrast, individuals of the second and third generations showed a progressive lowering of risk by between four- and five-fold.[79] Yet despite this lowered risk, third-generation Chinese immigrants were still 10 times more likely to develop NPC than the co-resident Caucasian population. These findings are an important first step towards our goal, that of disentangling the influence of nature (genetically endowed risk) from that of nurture (lifestyle-associated risk) on the chances of developing NPC. Strictly speaking, the lessons learned apply only to NPC as seen in Cantonese people but, by inference, they may well also be relevant to incidence of the tumour in other intermediate-risk populations. What we learn from the migrant studies is that genetic and lifestyle factors both play an important role in determining the risk of developing NPC. The falling incidence of disease in the locally born second and third generation individuals was attributed to the gradual dilution of the Cantonese lifestyle; however, the fact that these individuals were still much more likely to develop the disease than their non-Chinese compatriots was taken as strong evidence of an inherent genetic risk.

Interestingly, these findings are to some extent mirrored by the most recent studies on NPC incidence within South East Asia itself. Up to at least the year 2000, incidence rates in urban populations in mainland China had remained at their historically high levels. However, in places such as Hong Kong and Singapore, where the previous 50 years of economic development have inevitably diluted out the traditional Cantonese lifestyle, there are hints that NPC incidence is slowly beginning to fall. What's more, that trend is particularly apparent in the number of patients presenting at the younger end of the tumour's age range, in other words patients born later during the period of economic development, and therefore more likely to have experienced its lifestyle-changing effects.

It is one thing to know that lifestyle is important in determining NPC risk among Cantonese people, and quite another to determine what the important lifestyle factors might be. That problem had long fascinated John Ho in his day-to-day work with patients in Hong Kong. Ho was struck by the frequency with which he was diagnosing NPC in the 'boat people', a minority population of fisher-folk who for many generations had lived on sampans in Hong Kong harbour and were part of a wider community of boat dwellers stretching all the way from Hong Kong up the Pearl River delta to the city of Guandong (previously called Canton). His impression turned out to be correct—statistics released in 1972 showed that NPC incidence among these boat people was almost double that of the Hong Kong

Chinese population. Ho wondered if this could be caused by some aspect of their particular lifestyle. Others had already pointed out that the anatomical site where NPC first develops, in a specialized area at the rear of the nasal passages known as the Fossa of Rosenmuller, is exactly where any small particles present in inhaled air, particularly in smoke, become lodged. However, in the case of the boat people, smoke exposure seemed an unlikely explanation because they traditionally cooked, and burnt their incense sticks, not in a confined space, but on deck in the open air. Instead, Ho fixed on another aspect of Cantonese culture that was particularly marked in boat people, that is the omnipresence of salted fish in their diet. This was not just the type of salted fish people in the West might imagine—to get the best taste and aromatic flavour, freshly caught fish were dropped live, innards and all, straight into the pickling jar. Ho predicted correctly that such a food source would be high in N-nitrosamines, chemicals that were known to be potentially carcinogenic. On this basis, he speculated that salted fish in the diet, and especially the boat people's practice of weaning their infants onto salted fish very early in life, was the main environmental factor contributing to the high NPC incidence seen in the Cantonese.

It is notoriously difficult to formally prove any specific association between a dietary component and cancer. Such attempts typically involve retrospective analysis of the dietary histories of cancer patients versus matched controls and, as such, are subject to the inevitable frailties of human memory. Nevertheless, several studies among Chinese and some other South East Asian peoples have produced data consistent with Ho's theory linking salted fish consumption in childhood to increased NPC risk, and his ideas retain strong purchase to this day. Interestingly, they may also be relevant to tumour risk in another people of Mongol origin, albeit one far from South East Asia, the Inuits of Greenland. These people, with a diet high in both fresh and dried fish, have an intermediate incidence of NPC and are also uniquely susceptible to a salivary gland carcinoma which, because it is also EBV-positive and has the same appearance as NPC, seems to be a closely related variant of the nasal tumour. Dietary factors may also play a role in other populations with intermediate NPC incidence, for example in Tunisia, where certain traditional spices have been found to be rich sources of nitrosamines.

However, diet is very unlikely be the whole story in every context. Thus there are epidemiological studies in other intermediate risk South East Asian populations that link increased NPC risk with heavy cigarette smoking or with prolonged occupational smoke exposure. Perhaps most interesting in this respect are the observations of Clifford in Kenya, where NPC is well known, but where incidence rates are still poorly defined. As an ENT surgeon in Kenya in the 1960s and 1970s, Clifford noticed that NPC patients were not coming from the low-lying equatorial regions where Burkitt Lymphoma was endemic, but from the much cooler highland areas. These geographical differences could not be explained by genetics since the same peoples occupied both climatic zones, so the difference must be environmental. A visit to the cool highlands immediately suggested an explanation. For warmth, the highland people lived in poorly ventilated huts where fires burnt most of the day and for many hours of the night, producing soot that proved to be rich in aromatic hydrocarbons, a classic source of carcinogens.

Looking at all the evidence, there are very strong grounds for saying that lifestyle does impact on NPC risk and this most likely occurs through aerosol exposure to environmental carcinogens of one kind or another. These cofactors may be as various as human cultures themselves, but there is nevertheless a unifying concept, namely exposure to chemicals which either directly or indirectly damage DNA. In so doing they can introduce mutations that push a cell one step along the road from normality to malignancy.

* * *

Lifestyle is important, therefore, but the very marked geographic differences in NPC incidence worldwide (Figure 13) cannot be wholly explained by differences in lifestyle. It seems that some human population groups are inherently more susceptible to NPC than others

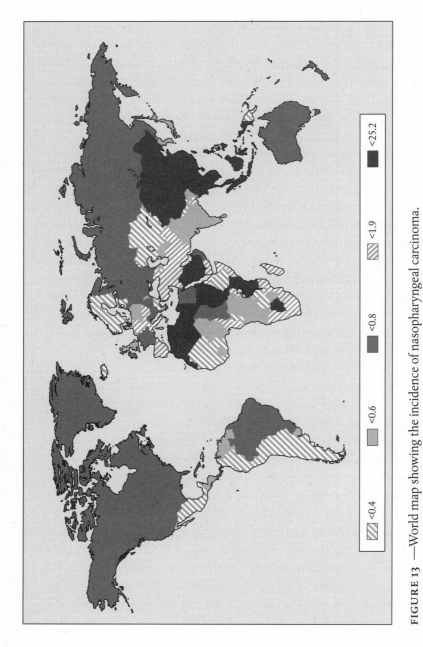

FIGURE 13 —World map showing the incidence of nasopharyngeal carcinoma. (Note that this Map uses disease incidence from national statistics and so, for China, does not show the large variation of incidence within the country, from low in the north to high in the south.)

and, as the migration studies show, carry that susceptibility with them down the generations. The influence of genetics is again apparent when one looks at tumour incidence in families within susceptible populations. An individual's risk of developing the tumour is significantly higher if another family member has previously been affected; indeed, up to 10 per cent of Chinese patients with NPC will report having a relative who has suffered the same disease.

Work on the genetics of NPC susceptibility naturally began with, and remains largely focused on, the Chinese population. However these investigations were immediately beset by a problem. NPC incidence within the vast land mass of China itself differs strikingly with geography, incidence rates being very low (less than 2/100,000/year) in the north and west, increasing to intermediate values as one moves south and east to the central provinces bordering the Yangtse River, and finally reaching the highest levels (more than 20/100,000/year) in the southern provinces of Guandong, Guangxi, and the island of Hainan. Such geographic differences do not sit easily with the idea of a genetically determined risk because the vast majority of China's population are considered to have a common ancestry, the so-called Han people, an ethnic group native to East Asia who subsequently became dominant through most of China's land mass. But in reality this view is greatly oversimplified. Migration from the Han heartland, and inter-marriage with different aboriginal peoples, have over centuries led to significant diversification within the Han family. This is apparent, not just from cultural traits such as custom and language, but also from recent genetic profiling, which has shown a gradual north–south gradient of genetic change in contemporary Chinese populations that matches the course of Han migration. And even in the south, there is ethnic diversity that again relates to NPC risk, with incidence of the tumour in people who speak the Guangzhou (Cantonese) dialect being up to two-fold greater than in the Hakka, Hokkien, and Chiu Chau dialect groups. Interestingly, among the many Southern Chinese who have migrated to Singapore, Cantonese speakers are again at higher risk than the other dialect groups. However, those differences are minor when one compares Singapore Chinese with the native Malays and with the city's Indian community, in whom NPC incidence is respectively 6-fold and 30-fold lower than that of the local Cantonese. Thus, the microcosm of Singapore graphically illustrates how, within a single city, genetic inheritance dominates NPC risk.

The dramatic increase in NPC cases seen among Han people when one moves from north-west to south-east within China suggests that susceptibility to the tumour originally lay within an aboriginal population, living in the south coast region, with whom the migrating Han intermarried. Successive waves of migration in different localities and at various times over the past 2,000 years have given rise to the different dialect groups seen in the south today, each with their own acquired level of NPC risk. But who might these original inhabitants have been? Ancient Chinese texts refer to groups collectively known as the 'Bai Yue' people as occupying a wide swathe of the coastline bordering the South China Sea. Eventually their state was overrun by Han invaders from the north. So while Bai Yue people continued to survive in their ancestral domain, they gradually lost their common identity: some were absorbed by the Han and others became disparate minority peoples. Now, if we look at the make-up of the Chinese population today, one of the minority people considered to be closest to the Bai-Yue are the Zhuang, a group to whom the 'boat people' of the Pearl River delta are thought to be related. Though the boat people remained in their ancestral homeland, they largely retained a separate identity because, for centuries, imperial decrees had forbidden them from living inland or from marrying Han people, apparently as retribution for their military resistance to colonization in times past. So, by force of circumstance, the Zhuang and their offshoot, the boat people, give us a glimpse of the aboriginal population who were in the region of present-day Guandong/ Guanxi before the Han arrived. And intriguingly, like today's boat people, the Zhuang minority also has an unusually high incidence of NPC.

This is the background to a hypothesis, recently put forward by Joseph Wee and colleagues in Singapore[80] that links Bai-Yue ancestry and NPC risk. They noticed that anthropologists had described a number of cultural practices shared between minority groups such as the Zhuang in China and aboriginal peoples in seemingly far-distant South East Asian locations. These included the Dayaks and Kayans of Borneo, the Bataks of Sumatra, and certain aboriginal people of Taiwan and the Phillipines. Even more interestingly, there were cultural parallels with isolated ethnic groups in the north-east of India, notably the Nagas and Manipurians, whose oriental features clearly distinguish them from the rest of the Indian population. Wee's striking insight was that all these groups, sharing cultural practices but physically separated across thousands of miles, were also distinguished by unusually high rates of NPC, often higher than those observed for Cantonese people in Guandong and Guangxi. He suggests that each of these are descendants of a Bai-Yue population that has been fragmented by conquest, forced migration, and the exigencies of history, yet each still carries the genes imposing high NPC risk.

If susceptibility to NPC is indeed written in the genes, what might such susceptibility genes be? When that question was first framed in the early 1970s, knowledge of genetic differences between individuals in a single population, and between populations, was primitive compared to what we know today. However, there was one set of genes which were well known to show surprising variability (referred to as polymorphism), the histocompatability leukocyte antigen (HLA) genes. These act like a barcode to distinguish one person from another, and make proteins, the HLA antigens, that likewise differ between individuals. Indeed, it is these differences that make it so difficult to transplant organs successfully between unrelated individuals because the recipient's immune response will react to the foreign HLA antigens on the transplanted organ and reject it. Knowing a person's 'HLA' or 'tissue type' is therefore crucial for successful transplant surgery. It so happened that, in 1970, the World Health Organization (WHO) established the Immunology Research and Training Centre in Singapore, housing the first HLA typing facility in any non-Caucasian country. The HLA laboratory was led by a young medical geneticist, Malcolm Simons. This brought Simons into contact with Professor Shanmugaratnam, Director of Singapore's Cancer Registry and the doctor whose work on NPC incidence on the Chinese, Malay, and Indian ethnic groups in that city had been so influential in highlighting the importance of genetic risk. As things turned out, it was a match made in heaven: HLA meets NPC.

So it was that work began in Singapore comparing the HLA types of NPC patients of Chinese ethnicity with that of the local Chinese community as a whole. The results looked very interesting. Certain HLA antigens, either singly or in specific combinations, were more frequently present in NPC patients than in controls, and therefore appeared to be associated with increased risk. Conversely, some other HLA antigens were seen less frequently in patients, and were therefore associated with reduced risk.[81] Fast forward 40 years to the present day and the work has become much more sophisticated. The genetics of susceptibility to almost all diseases with a familial association, including NPC, are complex and typically involve multiple genes spread throughout the genome. Each of these genes might vary slightly in sequence between different individuals and each variation might have a very small effect on disease risk: as a result, the genetic susceptibility of any single individual to any particular disease will be determined by the sum of all those effects. Disentangling genetic susceptibility, therefore, requires massive genome-wide studies on large numbers of patients and controls. Such work, now moving at a furious pace as a result of the revolution in DNA-sequencing technology, is well under way. But so far, as applied to NPC, such studies have only been sufficiently powerful to locate the region harbouring the strongest association with tumour risk. Across the whole human genome, this turns out to be the region on chromosome 6 where the HLA gene complex is found.

So Simons and Shanmugaratnam had indeed been on the right track all those years ago. What's more, while the significance of their original findings was not clear at the time, a link between HLA gene identity and NPC risk now makes sound biological sense. It turns out that HLA genes have very important immunological functions. Among these is their role as central controllers of the immune response to virus infections. In fact, over millions of years of human evolution, the need to cope with infections from many different viruses has been one of the main forces driving HLA genes to become so variable, both within individual ethnic groups and between groups. So, while susceptibility to most forms of human cancer bears no relation to HLA type, it is entirely understandable that susceptibility to a virus-associated cancer, in this case NPC, should show exactly such an association. Interestingly, the two HLA genes whose combination is most strongly associated with increased NPC risk in Southern Chinese, A*0207 and B*46, have only ever been found in people of South East Asian origin. The fascinating possibility is that these particular genes were present within the original Bai-Yue people and entered into the gene pool of present-day Southern Chinese by inter-marriage.

* * *

The past few pages have taken the reader through stories of salted fish in Hong Kong, smoke-filled huts in Kenya, the history of human migrations in South East Asia, and the intricacies of the HLA gene complex. These give us a glimpse of how both nurture (lifestyle) and nature (genetic identity) can influence an individual's chances of developing NPC. Now we must add the third essential ingredient into the mix, EBV. The virus is associated with all cases of this cancer worldwide, and in each case the virus genome is present in every tumour cell carried as a circular mini-chromosome, just as it is in Burkitt Lymphoma. In addition, researchers have found that, within any one NPC tumour, every cell carries a circular EBV mini-chromosome of exactly the same size, a unique marker showing that the tumour has arisen from a single virus-infected epithelial cell.[82]

The probability of all this occurring by chance is infinitesimally small. So it seems almost certain that EBV is one essential link in the chain of events causing NPC. But how does it work, when does it work, and what exactly are the other links in the chain?

Because NPC is an epithelial cell tumour, it showed that the virus which everyone had previously thought to only infect lymphocytes, could sometimes find its way into epithelial cells. But for many years it was not clear if this was a rare accident or if the virus actually infected epithelial cells as part of its normal lifecycle in the body. The answer came in the mid-1980s, not from a laboratory working on EBV but from a quite unexpected source. The husband and wife team John and Deborah Greenspan were clinical researchers at the University of San Francisco Dental School. San Francisco was the epicentre of the 1980s US AIDS epidemic and, as oral surgeons, the Greenspans were encountering increasing numbers of AIDS patients with mysterious rough, wart-like growths in the mouth, usually on the side of the tongue, lesions they called 'oral hairy leukoplakia'. Since the AIDS retrovirus, HIV, profoundly weakens the immune system, particularly the T lymphocyte-mediated responses that control virus infections, it seemed very likely that these warty lesions would be caused by a members of the human wart virus family, the papillomaviruses. Indeed, the Greenspans did find that these lesions were sites where a virus was replicating in the outer layers of epithelial cells, exactly as a papilloma virus would do. But, to their great surprise, this was not a papilloma virus: it was EBV.[83]

The message was clear. EBV is not only able to infect oral epithelial cells but also can replicate in them, producing new infectious virus particles in the process. Furthermore, such infections were not just a peculiarity of HIV infection. Identical lesions were later found in individuals, such as transplant patients, whose immune system had been compromised by immune-suppressive drugs. In both situations immune suppression was magnifying what was very likely going on unnoticed in the oral epithelium of healthy

EBV-infected people. This finding helped to explain why, from the early days of EBV research, it had been possible to detect infectious EBV at low levels in the mouth washings of some healthy virus carriers. How the virus behaved in the body of healthy carriers had always been something of a mystery; now at least things were becoming a little clearer. It appeared that, while the lymphocyte system harboured the virus for life in silent (latent) form, it could occasionally release a small fraction of this virus to allow replication in epithelial cells in the oral cavity, producing infectious particles that could be passed on in saliva to another person. As methods for detecting the virus became ever more sensitive, low-level virus shedding in saliva was often detected in healthy virus carriers. But crucially, it was not possible to find any evidence of infection at the site in the nasopharynx where NPC develops. Even in the high-risk Cantonese population, the only time EBV was found in nasal washings or samples of nasopharyngeal tissues was as a latent infection of tumour cells, either in patients who already have early stage NPC or in a few very rare individuals where pre-cancerous lesions have been caught in the act of converting to NPC. So entry into nasopharyngeal cells must be very rare but, when the virus does get there, it is dangerous.

As with many cancers, converting a normal nasopharyngeal epithelial cell to full malignancy involves multiple steps that may well accumulate over a period of decades. Unfortunately, we know little about the order of events in NPC, mainly because it has been so difficult to find precancerous lesions that represent staging posts on the journey. However, going back to the studies on lifestyle-associated risk, these strongly suggest a key role for chronic exposure to environmental carcinogens from early life, perhaps beginning in infancy. Inhaled carcinogens can cause DNA damage in nasopharyngeal cells, eventually leading to genetic changes that promote cell growth and survival, generating a pool of long-lived daughter cells already on the way towards malignancy. What those genetic changes might be was first addressed by Dolly Huang, a founder member of John Ho's research team in Hong Kong, and has been pursued by many laboratories since.[84] The changes in NPC are more numerous and more complex than in Burkitt Lymphoma, and no single gene shows the same consistent association with the tumour as the c-myc oncogene enjoys with Burkitt cells. However some changes occur sufficiently often in NPC to warrant special attention. First, duplication of particular sequences on the long arm of chromosome 11 implies a role for a key oncogene identified at the duplicated site. Conversely, frequent loss of genetic material from the short arms of chromosomes 3 and 9 suggests the importance of losing or silencing particular growth-controlling genes present at those sites. An intriguing recent finding gives an important clue as to how such cellular genetic changes and EBV infection might combine in the course of NPC development. When the virus is introduced into normal nasopharyngeal epithelial cells in the laboratory, the virus genome is quickly lost and the infection dies out. However, when these normal cells are genetically altered to mimic some of the changes seen in NPC, then the cells can retain the virus genome and support a latent infection.[85] In the body, therefore, if nasopharyngeal epithelial cells in which such genetic changes have occurred are then by chance exposed to EBV, there is a greater risk that the virus will be retained and a focus of EBV-positive, pre-cancerous cells established.

To understand how the virus might then increase the chances of such cells developing into NPC, it was important to know which viral proteins were being made in the tumour. As mentioned above, the EBNA immunofluorecence test had already shown that the same EBNA1 protein as seen in Burkitt Lymphoma cells was also present in the epithelial tumour. However, this was not all. As we shall see in the next chapter, developments in the mid-1980s provided the tools to look at EBV protein expression much more carefully and, using these approaches, two other proteins were also often detected in NPC. These were the latent membrane proteins LMP1 and LMP2, so called because of their known association with the cell membrane. Their presence became especially significant when researchers found that LMP1 could maintain epithelial cells in an undifferentiated or poorly differentiated state, like that seen in the tumour, while LMP2 could promote their growth. Both effects would move these cells further along the path to malignancy. What else happens between EBV infection of the pre-cancerous cell and final emergence of the tumour is simply not clear, but the rarity with which EBV-positive pre-cancerous lesions have been found suggests that, once the virus has appeared on the scene, progression to full malignancy may be quite rapid. EBV infection may not be the final link in the chain but all the available evidence suggests that it is an essential link—without EBV there would be no NPC.

* * *

The realization that EBV's association with cancer is not limited to Burkitt Lymphoma but includes a second, quite different malignancy, NPC, was a major turning point. It showed that the virus's oncogenic potential was not just limited to B lymphocytes, but also included epithelial cells, the cell type which in normal circumstances was only used for producing infectious virus. The search for more EBV-associated epithelial cancers was on. But perhaps surprisingly, tumours of oral and tongue epithelium, which were the cells most likely to be naturally infected with the virus, were found to be EBV-negative, as were various other epithelial tumours in the head and neck area. The only exception was the occasional EBV-positive cancer of salivary gland epithelium seen in the Inuit people, but this was widely considered to be a rare variant of the nasopharyngeal tumour to which the Inuit were also susceptible. It seemed that EBV's connection with epithelial tumours had begun and ended with NPC. This remained the settled view for many years, yet the story was to have an unanticipated and very significant postscript. The nasopharyngeal and salivary tumours shared a quite characteristic feature, with large numbers of non-malignant lymphocytes infiltrating the tumour mass. This caught the attention of two US pathologists, Lawrence Weiss and Darryl Shibata, who were aware that tumours with a similar NPC-like appearance were occasionally seen elsewhere, notably in a very small subset of cases of gastric carcinoma. Working with colleagues in Japan, they collected gastric carcinomas of this particular rare type and found that they were indeed frequently EBV-positive.[86] Even more surprisingly, 10 cases of the more common (non-NPC-like) gastric carcinomas had been included as controls in the same study, and in one of these the malignant cells were also EBV-positive. Not for the first time in the EBV story, a study's control samples had thrown up an unexpected and important result. In this case, it led to a wider screening of stomach cancers that confirmed the virus' association, not just with the rare NPC-like cases, but also with a fraction of tumours of the more common type.[87] It is clear that EBV is present as a latent infection in some 2 to 10 per cent of gastric carcinomas in countries right across the globe. While the full significance of these findings still has to be explored, based on what we now know about the virus it seems very unlikely to be an innocent by-stander in these tumours. On the contrary, it suggests that, if by chance EBV infects a gastric epithelial cell that is already en route to malignancy, then the infection can complete the process. As we shall see from the global figures in chapter 8, both NPC and the virus-positive subset of gastric carcinomas are now recognized as major contributors to the overall burden of EBV-associated cancers worldwide. We have come a long way since 1966, when the first hint of a connection between EBV and a cancer of epithelial origin was met with such widespread incredulity.

6

New EBV Diseases:
An accident of nature,
an accident of medicine

In 1974 we stood on the brink of the second decade of the EBV story looking at an uncertain future. The presence of the virus in Burkitt Lymphoma and NPC cells was well documented. However, many continued to doubt the significance of these associations because the two tumours arose in quite different cell types and there was no coherent view on what the virus' role might be. While these questions raged, one thing was already clear: if the virus did indeed cause cancer in rare individuals, then explaining how that happened would be very difficult when so little was known about the virus infection in normal healthy people. If EBV was such a dangerous virus, how was it normally kept under control?

Part of the answer lay in understanding how the immune system responds to a virus that strikes at the heart of the body's defences, invading cells of the immune system itself. Let's begin by going back to the one disease known to be caused by EBV, infectious mononucleosis (glandular fever). Patients with that disease have just become infected for the first time and have massive numbers of 'atypical mononuclear cells' in the blood. Since EBV naturally infected B lymphocytes and transformed their growth in the laboratory, it was widely assumed that these atypical cells must be virus-transformed B lymphocytes. Then, in the early 1970s, new markers of lymphocyte identity came along and turned that assumption on its head. These cells were not infected B lymphocytes at all: they were uninfected T lymphocytes that were activated and seemed to be part of a massive immune response *against* the infection. But there was a problem with this interpretation: if this was a genuine immune response to the virus, it seemed extraordinarily large. T lymphocyte responses were known to be specific to the incoming virus, and so one type of virus could only activate a tiny fraction of the body's total T lymphocyte population, just the few cells that had the right receptors to recognize that particular virus. However, in infectious mononucleosis patients, most of the T lymphocytes in the blood were activated, and their total numbers were 5 or 10 times the normal levels. It was very hard to believe that the tiny fraction of EBV-specific T lymphocytes in the body had divided to produce these massive numbers. Yet, as later work showed, this was precisely what had happened. The T lymphocyte response seen in infectious mononucleosis was indeed specific for EBV, but it was expanded to a size never seen before with any other virus.

Once the acute phase of infectious mononucleosis is over and the virus is under control, most of these highly activated T cells simply die away because their job is done. But here's another paradox. Despite being so large, the T lymphocyte response to EBV never completely clears the virus from the body. Whenever anyone becomes infected, whether they develop infectious mononucleosis or not, some EBV-infected B lymphocytes always survive, and the virus is then carried for life. A fine balance has been struck between virus and host, one that allows this potentially dangerous infection to persist without threatening the life of its host. To achieve persistence, the virus is carried as a silent (latent) infection in a small fraction of B lymphocytes, typically between 1 and 100 cells in every million, the exact number varying between individuals but being surprisingly stable over time in any one individual. These latently infected cells circulate around the body anonymously, avoiding attention by adopting the lifestyle of the B lymphocyte population as a whole. However, given the right cues, these cells can became active again, switching to make infectious virus. This virus can pass either to other B lymphocytes that then become growth-transformed, or to epithelial cells in the mouth and throat that become miniature factories of infectious virus shedding. In most individuals, reactivated infections of this kind typically come and go over the course of a lifetime without ever causing symptoms. But this happy co-existence is absolutely dependent on the host immune system being well armed against the virus and keeping it in check. Thus, as soon as the virus re-emerges from its hiding place, EBV-specific T lymphocytes act to contain that re-emergence and prevent it reaching dangerous levels.

If we now turn to the new diseases indicated in the title of this chapter, both of these arise when disorders of the immune system occur and disturb the happy co-existence described above. The first is an accident of nature, that is, a disease restricted to individuals with a rare genetic mutation affecting their immune response; the second is an accident of medicine—a disease that appears when for medical reasons the immune response is deliberately impaired. As with so many new developments in the EBV field, the door to greater understanding was opened by inquisitive clinicians responding to the challenge of a disease which was not in the medical textbooks.

* * *

The accident of nature is 'fatal infectious mononucleosis'. This sounds like a contradiction in terms, given the classical description of infectious mononucleosis as a self-limiting disease. However that picture changed radically in 1974 and 1975 when three independent reports, all from the US, were published, describing primary EBV infections with fatal consequences. The first report[88] came from Columbus, Ohio where, in April 1972, doctors encountered a 16-year-old boy with a 10-day history of fever and the first signs of liver damage. He was diagnosed with infectious mononucleosis on the basis of a positive heterophil antibody test and the presence of atypical lymphocytes in the blood. However, the disease progressed rapidly and the boy died of liver failure within eight days of admission. The autopsy showed massive infiltration of activated lymphocytes throughout the tissues. Blood and tissue samples, sent to the Henles in an effort to confirm the original diagnosis, gave intriguing results. The patient had remained EBV antibody-negative through-out his illness, yet had clearly succumbed to EBV infection because his lymph glands contained high levels of EBV genome and lym-phocytes producing herpesvirus particles could be seen in the elec-tron microscope. At first this looked like a complete failure of the virus-specific immune response, though in retrospect it was never clear how many of the activated cells were virus-infected B lym-phocytes and how many might have been reactive T lymphocytes. This one case was sufficiently interesting in its own right, but the really important insight came from tracing the boy's family his-tory. Three male cousins, all on the mother's side of the family, had died of acute illnesses with very similar symptoms. Two of these were recent cases, from 1968 and 1969, and both had been found to be heterophil antibody-positive, while a third case went back to 1948, when it had been recorded as an acute leukaemia. Given this fascinating history, Henle and colleagues rightly concluded that the family had 'a genetically determined defect in the host response to the virus'.

These findings were quickly followed by other reports, from Worcester Massachussetts,[89] and from Michigan,[90] of families in which young boys had presented with rapidly progressing infectious mononucleosis-like infections of the kind described above. In both studies, however, other boys in these same kindreds had presented with different symptoms, being diagnosed either with an immune deficiency, characterized by a general inability to mount effective anti-body responses ('hypogammaglobulinaemia'), or with a lymphoma. This suggested that the genetic defect, though most obviously present-ing as fatal infectious mononucleosis, was more far-reaching in its effects. It was the leader of the Worcester study, David Purtilo, who first drew attention to the different presentations of this immune deficiency, and it was he who subsequently raised awareness of the condition, not least by giving it a memorable name, 'Duncan's disease', after the family described in his report.

That publicity helped to identify more Duncan-like families and, within three years of setting up an international registry for the disease, Purtilo had records of 100 affected boys in 25 kindred worldwide.[91] Of the first 100 cases, 75 had presented with severe infectious mononucleosis following primary EBV infection. Many of these boys died during the acute disease, but some survived, only to be later diagnosed, in a few cases, with antibody deficiency or lymphoma. Curiously, another 25 boys had no history of infectious mononucleosis when they first went to hospital, but presented with antibody deficiency or lymphoma. Furthermore, in some cases these conditions must have developed before EBV infection because a few of the affected boys later succumbed to acute infectious mononucleosis. All three disease presentations appeared to be independent consequences of the same underlying immune deficiency. Of the three, only the mononucleosis-like disease was brought on by EBV infection; however, that was not only the most common presentation but also the most dangerous.

One of the most fascinating features of the condition was the very marked pattern of genetic inheritance within families. The defect was carried by females, but its effects were only apparent in half of their sons. This had all the hallmarks of inheritance via the female sex-determining chromosome, the X-chromosome. Duncan's disease was therefore re-christened more correctly as 'X-linked lymphoproliferative syndrome', a name usually abbreviated to 'XLP'. Somewhere on one of the two X-chromosomes of female carriers was a damaged gene, and it was that X-chromosome that had been passed on to their affected sons. Finding that gene was essential, both to identify affected boys within such families before they fell ill and, more generally, to understand how damage to a single gene could have such dramatic but varied effects. There were soon some clues about the gene's position on the chromosome. By the early 1980s the XLP Registry had identified rare families where the defect was large enough to be visible under the light microscope as loss of material from one X chromosome. There were also very large XLP kindreds, for example one family with at least 19 affected males spanning three generations, which were invaluable for the genetic marker analysis available at that time. This narrowed things down to a particular part of the X chromosome, about 3 million base pairs in length, within which the elusive XLP gene must lie.

However, in the days before rapid human genome sequencing, finding the needle in this three million base pair haystack remained a mammoth task. Progress had to wait for improvements both in gene mapping technology and in the availability of sequence markers in that particular part of the genome. Finally, in 1998, two groups, one from Massachusetts General Hospital in Boston and the other from the Sanger Centre in Cambridge, UK, identified the affected gene at exactly the same time.[92,93] It contained a coding sequence of just 384 base pairs and was predicted to encode a small protein (we'll call it the XLP protein) just 128 amino acids in length. Every XLP patient had either lost this gene completely or had inherited a damaged version, and so they could not make the XLP protein. What the XLP protein actually does, and why it is important, could have remained a puzzle for several years had it not been for help from an unexpected source. Coincidentally, a group of researchers from Harvard Medical School had been looking for new proteins involved in pathways of communication between lymphocytes, and had found a small protein that was an important part of one such pathway. It was 128 amino acids in length and its coding sequence could be traced to a particular region of the X chromosome. Unwittingly they had discovered the XLP gene at the same time as the gene mappers, but by a different route and for a different reason.[94] This story shows how unpredictable science can be, and how synergy between apparently unrelated studies can suddenly transform a research field.

Identifying the XLP gene was indeed the key to understanding the disease. Before its discovery, the clinical symptoms of XLP, especially the antibody deficiency, had suggested that the problem lay with B lymphocytes. However, it turned out that the XLP gene was never active in those cells. It was only used in T lymphocytes and in another special subset of lymphocytes, called 'natural killer' or NK cells, which also help to control virus infections, usually at the very early stages of the immune response. XLP was therefore a disease where the problem ultimately lay with a defect in T lymphocyte and/or NK cell control. This made sense of some earlier findings from John Sullivan, a paediatrician who had originally worked with Purtilo and who carried out the closest study of XLP boys in the throes of primary EBV infection. Sullivan found that much of the damaging lymphocyte population in XLP was made up of activated T lymphocytes and NK cells.[95] In other words, XLP patients were making an even more exaggerated version of the response that in classical infectious mononucleosis patients brings the virus under control. However, that response seemed ineffective because despite its size it did not prevent increasing numbers of virus-infected B lymphocytes building up. This resulted in massive invasion of both infected and reactive lymphocytes into tissues such as the liver, and death from liver damage or coincidental bacterial infection.

At this point, it was still not clear why loss of the XLP protein made patients especially vulnerable to EBV and not to other common virus infections. The answer came first from researchers who found that, while NK cells from XLP patients were able to recognize and kill most types of virus-infected target cell, they could not recognize virus-infected B lymphocytes.[96] Later, T lymphocytes from XLP patients were shown to have the same defect as NK cells. In both cases the recognition of infected B lymphocytes depended upon an extra signal relayed within the reactive cell by the XLP protein; when the protein was missing, that extra signal did not get through and immune recognition failed. So EBV is lethal to XLP patients, not primarily because it is a cancer-associated virus but because it infects the one cell type that is invisible to the XLP immune response, the B lymphocyte. In just the same way, XLP patients suffer a generalized defect in antibody production because, for most antibody responses, the B lymphocytes making those antibodies require help from T lymphocytes. However, other XLP patients present with yet a third type of symptom, that is lymphoma, and this is not so easy to explain. These tumours are typically of B lymphocyte origin but, while some may be linked to EBV, many show no association with the virus. Perhaps in normal individuals, T lymphocytes and/or NK cells play an ongoing role in immune surveillance against B lymphocyte malignancy, and that surveillance is defective in XLP patients.

This brings us up to date with the XLP story, but one cannot end without reference back to David Purtilo, the person who did so much to promote interest in this genetic deficiency and champion research. David was a character, short in height but with the girth of a prize fighter and every bit as competitive. He was a highly skilled and knowledgeable pathologist, but had no formal training in laboratory research and proceeded to learn the trade on the job. As a result, some of his early publications are written in a narrative style that raised eyebrows among his more conservative scientific peers, who typically spend hours crafting and re-crafting their scientific reports. One story, not entirely apochryphal, will suffice—caught at home one evening with dictaphone in hand, he was asked if this was how he usually wrote his report's first draft. 'The first draft?' he replied with a mischievous grin. 'No, this is it, I'll check for spelling mistakes once it's typed up tomorrow, and then it's off to the journal.'

* * *

The second 'accident' promised in the chapter title begins in a completely different area of medicine, that of organ transplantation. For many years the holy grail of immunologists had been to understand the rules governing transplant rejection. We have already talked in chapter 5 about the HLA genes, and their variability between different individuals. We saw that there are good reasons why evolution has driven the HLA genes to diversify within the human population. However, such barcodes of personal identity are the curse of transplant medicine. Organ transplantation is easy between identical twins because they have exactly the same combination of HLA class I and class II genes, the perfect HLA match. But where there is a mismatch between donor and recipient, even if that affects only one or two of the 12 or more HLA genes making up each individual's type, it is enough to cause the recipient to reject the donor's organ as foreign. That rejection is brought about by T lymphocytes. Transplant doctors therefore aim to find a donor with as close an HLA match as possible, and then to lessen the chances of the transplanted organ being rejected by reducing the patient's immunity using immunosuppressive drugs. As a result, transplant medicine is a continual balancing act. Doctors have to find a level of immune suppression that is sufficient to prevent rejection, yet leaves enough immunity to deal with any infections that the patient might encounter.

Human organ transplantation began in the early 1960s, made possible by two advances that were later recognized by Nobel Prizes. These were the development by Joseph Murray (winner in 1990) of surgical methods for kidney transplantation and the discovery by Gertrude Elion and George Hitchings (winners in 1988) of immunosuppressive drugs that allowed graft survival. By 1963, over 200 kidney transplants had been performed worldwide, and by the late 1960s that number had risen more than 10-fold. Then, in 1968 and 1969, came the first reports of patients unexpectedly developing cancer within a year or two of receiving a transplant. Though the total number of such cases was small, the same phenomenon was being seen in several different centres in both North America and Europe. Transplant doctors were sufficiently concerned to create informal registries of cancer incidence in transplant patients worldwide and, by 1971, a definite trend was emerging. Cancer incidence was indeed increased among transplant recipients and, intriguingly, the cancers were of particular types, often types rarely seen in the general population. Most common were skin tumours, followed by lymphomas. The latter had unusual and often quite variable microscopic appearances, making them difficult to classify. Moreover, up to half of them presented at a very unusual site—the brain. If anything, 'post-transplant lymphomas' looked like a completely new category of tumour.

Many of the early reports describing these lymphomas were anecdotal. Numbers were small and their significance uncertain. However, by the mid-1970s, the registry set up by Thomas Starzl and Israel Penn in Denver, Colorado, US, had amassed more than 50 cases of lymphoma in a patient group of around 15,000. Based on such figures, the chances of lymphoma developing in a kidney transplant patient seemed to be at least 30 to 40-fold greater than in non-transplanted, healthy people.[97] Incidence rates remained broadly at these levels throughout the 1970s, during which time the drug discovered by Elion and Hitchings, azathioprine, was the immunosuppression of choice. While some side effect of the drug itself could not be entirely discounted, there were several other, more likely explanations for the appearance of post-transplant lymphomas. A foreign organ in the body naturally provided a source of chronic stimulation to the patient's immune system, and experiments in mice had shown that chronic immune stimulation could lead to lymphoma. What's more, this chronic stimulation might be made worse by the virus infections that often resurfaced in transplant patients. Herpesviruses were a particular problem in this respect, and one such, herpes simplex virus, was known to infect the nervous system, where tumours often developed. At the bottom of a long list of contenders came EBV, another herpesvirus, whose association with Burkitt Lymphoma also depended on a chronic stimulus, malaria.

The uncertainty was finally resolved in the early 1980s, hastened by a new set of circumstances. Worryingly, the introduction into clinical practice of a new immunosuppressive drug, cyclosporin, had caused a dramatic rise in post-transplant lymphoma incidence.

Unlike azathioprine, this new drug was specifically active against T lymphocytes, the cells that cause organ rejection, and expectations of its clinical effectiveness were high. However, these were quickly tempered by one of the first reports of its use in kidney transplant patients by the UK's leading transplant surgeon, Roy Calne. Of the first 35 patients receiving high doses of cyclosporin A, either alone or in combination with conventional immunosuppressive drugs, three had developed lymphoma within the first year of transplant. That report,[98] appearing in *The Lancet* in November 1979, not only raised alarm among transplant doctors but, more importantly, also brought the problem to the attention of a wider audience of clinicians and scientists. In January 1980 a leading group of heart transplant researchers from Stanford, US, reported that they too had seen a high incidence of lymphoma in their experiments with primates receiving cyclosporin post-transplantation.[99] Meanwhile, a team of virologists from the Public Health Laboratories in Cambridge, UK, obtained serum samples taken from Calne's patients before and after transplant and screened these for antibody responses to common herpesviruses. The results, published in March,[100] were very interesting. Compared to azathioprine-treated controls, cyclosporin treated patients were much more likely to have increased anti-viral antibody levels, particularly anti-EBV levels, suggesting that the new drug caused greater disturbance of the virus–host balance. Furthermore, one of the three lymphomas had arisen in a patient who had experienced primary EBV infection within the first month post-transplant, just three months before the tumour was diagnosed. Circumstance was beginning to point to EBV as having a hand in the disease process.

As it happened, the key finding was only months away, though no one would ever have predicted the chance encounter that made it possible. One of us, Dorothy Crawford, had spent three years as a Clinical Research Fellow in Epstein's laboratory in Bristol and had continued her interest in EBV after moving to the Immunology Department at the Royal Free Hospital in London. She had been on the lookout for fresh tissue from a post-transplant lymphoma for some time when she finally found one. She recalls: 'I just happened to overhear a conversation in a hospital lift between worried doctors from the kidney transplant unit. They were debating on how to treat their first post-transplant lymphoma patient.' This was just the break she had been hoping for. Fortunately, the pathologists had fresh tumour tissue for testing, and so Crawford and colleagues got to work. Amazingly, the tumour cells were EBNA-positive. The letter describing this work, published in *The Lancet* in June 1980,[101] showed for the first time that post-transplant lymphoma carried the EBV genome and that the virus was active in these tumour cells. Of course it was just a single case, but it alerted everyone to the possibility that EBV's associations with cancer might stretch beyond Burkitt Lymphoma and NPC.

In 1981 several more such reports appeared, the most important being from Douglas Hanto and colleagues at the University of Minnesota in Minneapolis, US. They described 12 cases of post-transplant lymphoma that had arisen among 1100 kidney transplant patients at their centre over the previous decade. Tumour samples were still available for molecular hybridization in eight cases and all proved to be EBV DNA-positive; furthermore, where cell preparations could be tested, the tumour cells were EBNA-positive.[102] The link to EBV was confirmed. Hanto's work also began to identify clinical patterns within the variable appearance of post-transplant lymphomas. Those that developed within the first year after transplantation often followed a recent primary EBV infection and tended to progress rapidly. Others developed later, up to 10 years post-transplant; these tended to present as a localized mass and grew more slowly, though still with a fatal outcome. Microscopically, these tumours were also variable in histological appearance and only some, usually the later onset tumours, had the uniform look of a classical lymphoma. This led to esoteric discussions among pathologists as to whether the early onset lesions could really be classified as malignancies. Eventually it was decided to re-christen all post-transplant lesions as 'post-transplant lymphoproliferative disease', but here we will stick with the shorter and simpler name, 'post-transplant lymphoma'.

The distinction drawn above between early and late onset lymphomas in kidney recipients will become important later on when discussion turns to what the virus is doing in these tumours. But right now we need to look at another branch of medicine that, by the 1980s, was experiencing its own outbreak of post-transplant lymphomas—bone marrow transplantation. This transplant technique was pioneered in the 1960s by Donnall Thomas working in Seattle, US, an achievement recognized by the 1990 Nobel Prize awarded jointly to Thomas and his counterpart in solid organ transplant surgery, Joseph Murray. As originally conceived, bone marrow from an HLA-matched donor could be used to reconstitute the entire blood cell (haemopoietic) system of patients who had received total body irradiation as treatment for acute leukaemia. The main concern, of course, was that the leukemia cells were not completely destroyed by the irradiation and so the disease would recur. What Thomas' team did not anticipate was the possibility that tumours might develop from cells within the bone marrow graft itself. Yet this was exactly what sometimes happened. In two unusual cases, originally described in *The Lancet* in 1971 and 1972, young girls had each received total body irradiation for acute lymphoblastic leukaemia, and then bone marrow transplants from their healthy HLA-matched brothers. In both cases the grafts were successful and the patients were disease-free until, two and four months later, they again developed lymphoblastic leukaemia. However, these malignant cells did not look like the original tumour, and indeed their chromosomes showed that they were male cells, derived from the bone marrow donors.[103, 104] Not surprisingly, the authors found it hard to explain such an unexpected result, and these donor-derived tumours were not further investigated at the time. But, with the benefit of hindsight, we can infer that these actually represent the first published cases of EBV-associated lymphoma following bone marrow transplantation.

The link between EBV and bone marrow transplant lymphomas was not formally demonstrated until a decade later in 1982, just after Crawford's and Hanto's reports on the kidney transplant cases. Again the key report came from Thomas' laboratory.[105] In this case a 5-year-old boy, treated for acute lymphoblastic leukaemia, received bone marrow from his sister who was partially HLA-matched. The boy then developed a rapidly fatal B cell lymphoma that was EBV DNA-positive and, by chromosome analysis, was shown to be derived from his sister's cells in the graft. Serum antibody testing showed the donor was an EBV carrier and so it seems likely that the tumour had arisen from virus-infected B lymphocytes that had been in the donor bone marrow preparation and had multiplied in the immune-compromised recipient. EBV was showing itself to be as much a problem in heavily immune-compromised bone marrow transplant patients as in kidney transplant recipients. Furthermore, as surgical techniques developed to allow organs such as the heart, lungs, or small bowel to be transplanted, the incidence of early onset lymphomas increased, reflecting the need for higher doses of immunosuppressive drugs to prevent rejection of these organs. Where the transplant recipient was a child, the risk was particularly great because many children were EBV-seronegative at the time of transplant and often acquired the virus from infected B lymphocytes, either within the transplanted organ itself or in accompanying blood transfusions. So they had to cope with the challenge of EBV infection without the advantage of having some immunological memory of the virus while at the same time receiving immunosuppressive drugs.

Identifying post-transplant lymphoma as a second EBV-associated B cell tumour immediately raised comparisons with Burkitt Lymphoma. Importantly, new research tools developed in the 1980s began to show just how different the two tumours were. First, post-transplant tumours often turned out to be 'oligoclonal', that is, they had arisen from a few (two, three or more) B lymphocytes, each of which had been converted to uncontrolled growth. This was very unusual and contrasted with Burkitt Lymphoma which, like almost all other forms of malignancy, was 'monoclonal', in other words, it arose from a single cell. Also, the early post-transplant tumours showed no evidence of any chromosome translocation of the kind seen in Burkitt Lymphoma cells. Everything suggested that there were fewer steps involved in the development of the post-transplant tumours and so more B lymphocytes completed the journey to uncontrolled growth. The most crucial difference, however, lay in the detail of viral activity in the two tumours. Knowing which viral genes, and therefore which viral proteins, were active in latently infected cells was key to progress in this as in many other areas of EBV research. Until the mid-1980s there were very few if any tools available to achieve this. Then the impasse was broken by one of the most important of all milestones in the EBV story: the sequencing of the virus genome.

The genomes of all herpesviruses are huge compared to most other virus types, and EBV is no exception. Within each tiny virus particle, there is a double-stranded DNA helix containing over 170,000 nucleotide base pairs whose sequence is unique to EBV. In 1964, when the virus was first discovered, determining that sequence must have seemed an impossibly distant goal. Methods for sequencing even the smallest piece of DNA had not yet been developed. Indeed, the first DNA sequence of any virus, a small monkey virus only 5000 base pairs in length, was not determined until 1978. Surely a herpesvirus sequence would be a step too far? Then fate took a hand in the person of Fred Sanger, a leading figure at the MRC Laboratory for Molecular Biology in Cambridge, UK, and one of the Nobel Prize-winning inventors of DNA sequencing technology. As luck would have it, in 1981 his team had just completed the 48,500 base pair sequence of a small virus of bacteria and was looking for the next challenge, something three or four times larger. EBV fitted the bill perfectly: its genome was about the right size, cloned fragments of that genome had already been made by colleagues in London, and, to cap it all, EBV was not just a convenient source of sequence-able DNA, it was a candidate human cancer virus. The EBV genome was both the largest to be sequenced at that time and also the first genome to be attempted with no prior idea of its gene content. Sanger handed leadership of the project to his deputy, Bart Barrell, charging the team to speed things up by improving sequencing technology and the means of sequence analysis as they went along. With an average of eight people on the project at any one time, the 172,282 base pair sequence of the B95.8 strain of EBV was determined to a high degree of accuracy within three years. Paul Farrell, the one member of the team who went on to build a career in EBV research, remembers 'writing a small postcard in the early 1980s which remained pinned on the notice board in Bart Barrell's office for several years. On this card I worked out pro rata with our progress on the EBV project, using the same technology, how long it would take Bart to sequence the human genome. The answer was 25,000 years!' Yet such was the pace of technological change over the next two decades, and the size of the international effort led in part from the newly formed Sanger Institute in Cambridge, UK, that the first human genome sequence was completed in 2001, a mere 24,980 years ahead of schedule.

Publication of the EBV sequence, in Nature in 1984,[106] marked a huge turning point. Up till then it had been possible to cut the genome into pieces and arrange those pieces back in order, but there was little idea of what genes each piece contained. Now one could see that the virus contained upwards of 80 genes, each with its own unique sequence, arranged along the full length of the genome. Understanding what role each of these genes played during the life cycle of the virus would be an immense long-term challenge. However, the immediate objective was clear: to identify the subset of genes involved in the virus' links with cancer. In that regard, there was a ready place to start. EBV's ability to transform B lymphocytes into permanent growth in the laboratory had always been its talisman, the best evidence of its potential to act as a tumour virus. Assuming that this same ability was likely to be at work in tumours, several laboratories had already begun studying the signatures of the virus' activity in transformed cells. Those signatures were the messenger RNAs that relay genetic information embedded in the DNA sequence of the virus and allow that information to be translated into the amino acid sequence of virus-coded proteins. Importantly, only a small number of messages, far fewer than the total coding capacity of the virus, were detectable in virus-transformed cells. That implied that only a small number of the virus' genes were active in transformation. Now, with the genome sequence at hand, it was possible to look along that DNA sequence to find the source of those messages and thereby find the virus' 'transforming' genes. This approach identified just eight protein-coding genes, spread out at different places along the genome. Each had its own unique sequence, from which one could infer the amino acid sequence of its protein product, making it possible to develop antibodies that would detect that protein specifically. This led in time to the identification of all eight 'transforming' proteins. One of these was EBNA1, the nuclear antigen first found in both Burkitt Lymphoma and NPC cells by immunofluorescence. But in addition, virus-transformed B lymphocytes also contained five other virus-coded nuclear antigens (christened EBNAs 2, 3A, 3B, 3C, and –LP) and the two latent membrane proteins LMP1 and LMP2.

Although it would take many years to work out how these eight proteins co-operate with one another to transform B lymphocyte growth, one thing was immediately clear. Finding all eight proteins together in an infected cell was a sure sign of a growth-transforming EBV infection. Crucially, this is exactly what was found in early onset post-transplant lymphomas, in stark contrast to Burkitt Lymphoma where, despite using the whole range of antibodies to latent proteins, only EBNA1 was detectable. The implication was clear: post-transplant tumours really were the direct consequence of EBV transformation events happening in the body. Furthermore, these tumours looked very much like the lymphomas that, years earlier, Anthony Epstein and George Miller had observed in owl monkeys and tamarins after infection with high doses of EBV. In those experiments, immunosuppressive drugs had increased the animals' susceptibility to lymphoma. Also, when re-examined using the new tools, these experimental lymphomas turned out to be oligoclonal, lacked obvious chromosomal aberrations, and expressed the full spectrum of EBV latent proteins.

With these findings in hand, it became easier to understand why transplant patients were at risk of lymphoma, and why that risk was greatest when immune impairment was most intense. Immuno-suppressive therapy was designed to inhibit the T lymphocyte system because cells of this type brought about organ rejection. However, T lymphocytes were also vital for keeping virus infections under control. Indeed, while these studies on post-transplant lymphomas were going apace, other work was showing that all healthy EBV-infected individuals had a powerful T lymphocyte surveillance system that specifically recognized EBV latent proteins. These T lymphocytes, it was argued, were continually looking for and removing EBV-transformed B lymphocytes if and when they arose. When that surveillance was weakened, virus-transformed cells would have more opportunity to survive and grow, and eventually some of them would make it through to produce post-transplant lymphoma. This hypothesis also had an interesting prediction: that the lesions arising in patients would remain susceptible to surveillance if T lymphocyte immunity were restored. In 1984, proof that this was indeed the case came from Thomas Starzl, one of the leaders in the field of solid organ transplantation. In an influential publication in The Lancet,[107] he reported that the lymphomas, whether arising at low incidence in his kidney transplant patients or at much higher incidence in his heart–lung transplant patients, frequently disappeared when immunosuppressive therapy was reduced. The realization that these EBV-positive lesions remained under immunological control was of major importance, not just for the clinical management of patients but also in a broader context. It identified post-transplant lymphomas as a prime model for the development of T cell-based therapies against cancer in general, a theme that we shall pick up later in chapter 8.

Before we leave this part of the story, let's set the record straight by adding an important caveat. As time passed, it became clear that not all post-transplant lymphomas fell into the neat picture painted above. So far we have been discussing early onset tumours, those arising either in bone marrow transplant patients before their immune competence is fully restored or in solid organ transplant patients within the first year post-transplant when their immuno-suppression is most intense. However, most solid organ recipients remain on low levels of immunosuppression for life and, as more patients were followed for longer times, it became clear that their lymphoma risk was now lower but still remained above that of the general population. Some of the late onset lymphomas seemed to be directly driven by the virus, just like the early onset tumours. Others are different and appear to have arisen by more complicated routes involving cellular genetic changes of various kinds. Some of these are still EBV-positive but express a more limited range of viral pro-teins, while others lack the virus altogether. Despite these caveats, the example of post-transplant lymphoma turned out to be hugely important. It showed that EBV infection could lead directly to a form of cancer in the virus' natural host. On this evidence alone, and with-out recourse to all of the virus' other tumour associations, EBV earned the right to be called a human tumour virus.

* * *

The accident of nature that is XLP and the accident of medicine that is post-transplant lymphoma are bound together in this chapter, both for chronological and scientific reasons. Chronologically, both appeared on the scene in the early 1970s under the title of new dis-eases. Of course XLP was 'new' only in the sense that it was being described for the first time in print, but must have occurred in rare families over millennia. By contrast, the lymphoma was genuinely novel, an unforeseen consequence of twentieth-century medicine and its use of immunosuppressive drugs. In terms of understanding EBV's links to malignancy, another important truth emerged. The virus was now causally linked with two very different tumours of B lymphocytes: Burkitt Lymphoma and post-transplant lymphoma. These two tumours arose in quite different circumstances and the virus' role in tumour development appeared to be different in the two situations. In Burkitt Lymphoma it was acting as a complement to the uncontrolled growth signals from a key cellular oncogene, c-myc; in post-transplant lymphoma the virus itself was the main driver of cell growth. From the 1980s onwards, reconciling these two different aspects of EBV's behaviour was to become a central theme of much research. Yet right from the start, as if to emphasize the complexity of the task, there came a turn of events showing that both types of tumour could arise in one type of patient.

In 1980 the first reports appeared of an outbreak of opportunistic infections among young gay men in San Franscisco. This heralded the appearance of another new disease, the acquired immunodeficiency syndrome, AIDS, and its causative agent the human immunodeficiency virus, HIV. Many of the symptoms of AIDS reflect the fact that HIV infects and destroys CD4 T lymphocytes, a cell type that is important in helping both antibody and T cell-mediated immune responses. This inevitably compromises the ability of a patient to deal with many resident infections, but the consequences were particularly interesting in the case of EBV. Already in the previous chapter we saw how lesions appearing in the mouths of AIDS patients allowed foci of EBV replication in epithelial cells to be visualized for the first time. Here we see how the HIV epidemic advanced our understanding of EBV-associated lymphomas.

While many HIV-infected patients first presented with pneumonia from opportunistic lung infections, others presented with particularly unusual types of cancer. Some of the most frequently seen cancers were a range of lymphoid tumours known collectively as the AIDS-lymphomas. One of these was a lymphoma that often presented in the brain, and typically involved patients in late-stage AIDS with profound T cell impairment. The parallels with post-transplant lymphomas were obvious, and indeed these tumours were almost exclusively EBV-positive and, where analysed, showed the same signatures of virus-driven lymphoproliferative lesions as the early post-transplant disease. But that was by no means the full story. Other HIV-infected patients were presenting with a tumour that looked remarkably like a different EBV-associated malignancy, Burkitt Lymphoma.[108] This was so unexpected as to seem fanciful. Up to that point, the Burkitt tumour had been a very rare disease in the US and, in any case, was usually seen in children. Yet, as luck would have it, the clinicians at the centre of the AIDS epidemic had a Burkitt expert on their doorstep. John Ziegler, who had been the first director of the Uganda Cancer Institute in Kampala in the 1960s and had spent more than a decade working on the tumour in its endemic form, had taken up a post at the University of California in San Francisco in the summer of 1981. Ziegler recalls that 'We were astonished that cases of Burkitt's lymphoma, some even presenting in the jaw like the African tumour, would suddenly appear in the AIDS patient population. It was Uganda redux, but this time in adult Americans in the setting of serious immune abnormalities. Patients started out with signs of immune stimulation and enlarged lymph nodes but quickly became immune suppressed.' To confirm that this really was Burkitt Lymphoma, later studies showed that all cases had the same chromosomal translocations as the African tumour. Furthermore, in contrast to the very low EBV-association rate shown by Burkitt Lymphoma in American children, some 30–40 per cent AIDS-associated cases were EBV-positive, and, where the virus was present, it behaved exactly as it does in cells of the African tumour, expressing only the EBNA1 protein.

The appearance of Burkitt Lymphoma as an AIDS-associated malignancy is especially important to this story. It is one example, of which there are many in science, where an observation that is completely unexpected, even contradictory, when first made eventually leads to a deeper understanding of its subject. One of the key lessons here came from the timing of the tumour's appearance. While the post-transplant-like lymphomas only developed in late-stage AIDS when the patient was profoundly immune-compromised, Burkitt Lymphomas typically developed early in the course of HIV infection while the patient was still relatively immune-competent. We now know that, although HIV is linked to immune suppression as the infection progresses and CD4 T lymphocyte function is lost, paradoxically the early phase of HIV infection is associated with persistent lymph gland enlargement and hyper-stimulation of B lymphocytes. It is in this early phase of the infection that Burkitt Lymphoma typically appears, just as one might expect if such hyper-stimulation increases the chances of cells acquiring one of the rare chromosomal translocations discussed in chapter 4. Where EBV is around to assist tumour development by complementing the effect of that chromosomal change, it duly will.

AIDS patients therefore provide a unique example in which two of the best known EBV-associated malignancies, post-transplant-like lymphoma of the immune-compromised and Burkitt Lymphoma, are seen within the same patient group. Clearly the events involved in the development of these two malignancies, and the circumstances that predispose to those events, are different. To emphasize those differences, in more recent years, as anti-viral drugs have been developed to contain HIV infection and delay the patient's progression to a profoundly immunosuppressed state, the incidence of the post-transplant-like tumour has markedly fallen, whereas that of Burkitt Lymphoma has not.

Today we have a better understanding of EBV's multi-faceted ability to cause disease. However, some lessons were already clear by the mid-1980s. Two decades of research were showing that EBV could contribute to malignant change in different ways, even within the same cell type, the B lymphocyte. If that were the case, might the next 10 years uncover even more virus-associated lymphomas?

7

Unexpected Arrivals: Hodgkin Lymphoma and the T/NK cell lymphomas

Thomas Hodgkin was born in London in 1798 into a devout Quaker family and maintained those religious ideals throughout a somewhat troubled life. In those days entry into the medical schools at Oxford and Cambridge was closed to Dissenters and so Hodgkin trained in Scotland, at Edinburgh University, before spending 12 years back in London as a lecturer at the newly established Guy's Hospital Medical School. There he pioneered the study of disease pathology and, in 1832, published the first description of a fatal condition involving progressive enlargement of the lymph glands that resembled, but he believed was different from, tuberculosis.[109] Such work would surely have been the springboard to a successful academic career had its true significance been immediately recognized. But circumstance, and Hodgkin's deep commitment to radical social reform, took him on another course and he spent the rest of his life alongside his close friend, the philanthropist Moses Montefiore, working as a champion of oppressed peoples both within Britain and abroad. He died on a visit to Palestine in 1866. We do not know whether he ever saw a report which had been published, again from Guy's Hospital, just one year earlier. The condition he first described had been re-discovered and, in a final act of good grace, given the eponym 'Hodgkin's Disease'.

Despite the attention a memorable name can bring, Hodgkin's Disease remained an enigma. Was it caused by an ongoing infection, akin to tuberculosis, or was its progressive spread within the lymph glands really the sign of a cancer? In Vienna one young pathologist, Carl Sternberg, took the former view; while another in Baltimore, US, Dorothy Reed, took the latter. We remember these names today because their reports, published in 1898 and 1902 respectively, gave the first detailed descriptions of Hodgkin's Disease tissues as seen under the microscope.[110,111] A variety of white blood cells made up the bulk of the swollen glands, but there were also some unusual giant cells, now called Reed-Sternberg cells, that seemed to be a signature of the disease. Later work was to show that these giant cells really are the malignant population and are surrounded by a large infiltration of non-malignant cells. So Dorothy Reed had been right. Hodgkin's Disease was indeed a form of cancer, albeit a very unusual one where the malignant cells, rather than being the majority population as in most cancers, make up just 1–2 per cent of the whole tumour mass. Interestingly, just as with Hodgkin's contribution to medical science, the significance of Reed's work was not recognized until much later, in this case long after she had left pathology out of frustration at the lack of academic prospects for women at that time.

The malignant nature of the Hodgkin's disease was finally clear but the next challenge, to identify the origin of the Reed-Sternberg cell, continued to defy researchers for almost the whole of the twentieth century. While ever more sophisticated markers were able to distinguish one type of normal cell from another, Reed-Sternberg cells would fit none of the neat categories: they appeared to be chimaeric, combining markers from quite different types of white blood cells. What's more, their small numbers in Hodgkin's Disease tissues meant that these malignant cells could not be prepared as a pure population for thorough investigation. Ultimately, the breakthrough came with the development in the 1990s of micro-dissection, a technique allowing individual cells to be picked out from slices of tumour tissue under a microscope. It was painstaking work, but in that way individual Reed-Sternberg cells could be isolated and their DNA analysed. In 1994 Ralf Kuppers and colleagues in Germany gained the first definitive evidence from the analysis of these cells' immunoglobulin gene sequences.[112] Reed-Sternberg cells had the genetic signature of B lymphocytes even though they had lost many conventional markers of their original identity during conversion from the normal to the malignant state. Moreover, within any one tumour, all the Reed-Sternberg cells carried the same unique immunoglobulin sequence, so they were all descendents of the first malignantly converted cell, the true sign of a monoclonal tumour. Thus the long-standing mystery had been solved. Hodgkin's Disease was a tumour of B lymphocyte origin and could legitimately be re-christened Hodgkin Lymphoma.

It is no accident that we have covered almost two hundred years of the history of Hodgkin Lymphoma without yet mentioning EBV. The two stories do indeed interconnect, but for a long time the idea of a causative link between virus and disease was viewed with justifiable scepticism. Even as late as 1990, some authoritative reviews on EBV's disease associations contained no reference to this lymphoma. However, people had long suspected that the disease had an infectious cause because of its unusual age-dependence. While the lymphoma occurs worldwide and risk increases with age in most populations, its incidence in the Western world is significantly higher than elsewhere, reflecting the added burden of a large number of cases appearing among young adults. Such a young adult peak of disease incidence was very unusual for a malignancy (Figure 14). Furthermore, when pathologists began to classify Hodgkin Lymphomas into distinct types based on the patterns of the infiltrating normal cells, most of these young adult cases were of one particular type, now called the nodular sclerosing, whereas most of the older age and the occasional childhood cases were of another—the mixed cellularity. This led to the idea that the young adult disease was a separate entity, perhaps linked to its own infectious agent. In addition its age distribu-

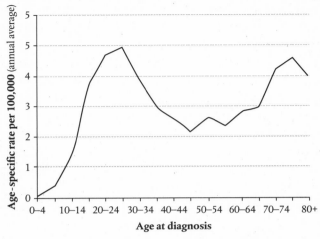

Source: Cancer Care Ontario (Ontario Cancer Registry, 2006)

FIGURE 14 Chart showing the age-related incidence of Hodgkin Lymphoma as seen in the developed world

tion was exactly what would be expected if the infectious agent was one that was usually acquired early in life but, in more affluent Western societies, was not acquired until later, when the chance of it causing disease might be greater. The parallels with EBV, where delayed primary infection causes infectious mononucleosis, were all too apparent.

The first study into a possible link between EBV and Hodgkin Lymphoma was carried out by the Henles who, working with George Klein's research team, looked at EBV antibody levels in patients presenting with the disease. Published in 1970, their work revealed a mixed picture.[113] Levels of EBV capsid and membrane antibodies were increased in the patient group compared to controls, but the differences were less consistent than seen with Burkitt Lymphoma or NPC patients and the mean values nowhere near as high. Furthermore, the young adult patients with nodular sclerosing-type tumours showed the least impressive elevations. That result, and subsequent work showing that antibody responses to other herpesvirus infections were also elevated in Hodgkin's patients, dampened any immediate enthusiasm for the idea that EBV might be causally related to the tumour. In fact, Hodgkin Lymphoma patients in general seemed to suffer a slight immunologic impairment affecting all T lymphocyte-mediated responses. So the heightened antibody levels appeared more likely to be a secondary effect, a response to the increased levels of virus infection that built up as a result of reduced T lymphocyte-mediated control. Interestingly, tests on samples retrieved from large population-based serum banks in the US found that some individuals who later developed Hodgkin Lymphoma had elevated EBV antibody levels several years beforehand, suggesting that the virus–host imbalance had been long-standing. But whether this pre-existing imbalance had anything to do with the disease process remained a matter of conjecture.

The only hint that a connection between EBV and the disease might still be worth pursuing came from two epidemiological studies published in 1974, based on large population records held in Denmark and in Connecticut, US. Both reported that patients with a history of infectious mononucleosis had a three to four-fold increased risk of developing Hodgkin Lymphoma over the following five years.[114,115] But it was not clear whether this increased risk was a direct result of acquiring EBV per se, or just a by-product of the profound immunological disturbance that the lymphoid system suffered during acute infectious mononucleosis.

By the early 1980s the link between EBV and two malignancies of B lymphocytes, Burkitt Lymphoma and post-transplant lymphoma, was well established. To most observers, the chances of that link extending to Hodgkin Lymphoma, then still a tumour of uncertain origin, seemed remote. Yet, if an idea has a grain of truth, the vast melting pot of clinical experience has an uncanny knack of producing rare cases that can keep the idea alive. One such case involved a family from West Virginia, US, in which, very unusually, a daughter had already died from an overwhelming infectious mononucleosis-like disease after primary EBV infection. Her 6-year-old brother then suffered a similar acute infectious mononucleosis but survived, only to progress within a year to develop classical Hodgkin Lymphoma.[116] But at the time this seemed more likely to be complete coincidence than evidence of any causal link with EBV. By contrast, a second case, described by Sibrand Poppema and colleagues in Groningen, the Netherlands, was firmer in its support for a viral role.[117] This involved a 69-year-old man who was receiving immunosuppressive therapy for allergic lung disease and suffered from an infectious mononucleosis-like illness, often called reactivated EBV infection. This took the form of recurrent bouts of lymph gland swelling that at first resembled an EBV-associated post-transplant tumour but later progressed to a lymphoma with the classical appearance of Hodgkin Lymphoma. What's more, the Reed-Sternberg cells in this tumour were clearly EBNA-positive. This was the first indication of EBV infecting Reed-Sternberg cells, exactly the kind of evidence that just five years earlier had sealed the link between EBV and post-transplant lymphoma.

It may seem surprising, but neither of these reports caused much of a stir at the time of their publication, in 1983 and 1985 respectively, and even today they are rarely cited. Both described unusual cases of Hodgkin or Hodgkin-like Lymphoma arising in patients who, for one reason or another, were severely immune compromised. As such, their relevance to Hodgkin Lymphoma as it arose in the general population seemed doubtful. It was left to others, using a different approach, to take the research forward. At the time Lawrence Weiss was working in Stanford, California, with Jeff Sklar, whose research group had already made important contributions to the study of EBV-associated lymphomas using immunoglobulin gene sequences as markers of clonality. Applying this approach to Hodgkin Lymphoma samples had already given some intriguing results. Certain samples contained immunoglobulin gene signals suggesting that a mono-clonal B lymphocyte population was present somewhere within the tumour mass. However, to argue that these signals actually came from the malignant Reed-Sternberg cells seemed a step too far; indeed, the work formally proving these cells to be B lymphocytes was still almost 10 years away. Another possibility was that the signals came from an expanded population of non-malignant B lymphocytes that was infiltrating the tumour, and the most likely explanation for such an expansion was that the cells were EBV-infected. For that reason Weiss and colleagues probed DNA from Hodgkin tumour samples to look for the EBV genome. Four out of 21 samples contained detectable EBV DNA; however, those four did not match the tumours that had immunoglobulin gene signatures of normal B lymphocyte expansion.[118] This unexpected result had a fascinating implication: that EBV was not present in the normal infiltrating B lymphocytes but that a subset of Hodgkin Lymphomas carried EBV in the malignant cells themselves.

That work, published in 1987, attracted much attention and led over the next three years to a flurry of reports from the Stanford group and others. These studies confirmed that EBV was linked to some, but not all, cases of Hodgkin Lymphoma. Key to this was the development of *in situ* hybridization techniques that could detect either virus DNA or a particularly abundant virus-coded RNA[119] present within individual cells. These proved that, in EBV-positive cases, the virus genome was actually present in the Reed-Sternberg cells and not in the normal cell infiltrate. Subsequently, staining such EBV-positive cases with specific antibodies showed that the virus was expressing three proteins in these tumour cells, EBNA1 (in the absence of the other EBNAs) and high levels of the two latent membrane proteins LMP1 and LMP2. This was different from the pattern of expression seen either in Burkitt Lymphoma or in post-transplant lymphoma. The message was again loud and clear: EBV behaved differently in different tumour types and, by inference, very likely contributed in different ways to the disease process.

With the tools now in place to detect the virus in archival collections of Hodgkin Lymphoma specimens, events moved swiftly. The first study of LMP1 staining of Reed-Sternberg cells had reported that

EBV was linked to the majority (>90 per cent) of cases studied of the mixed cellularity type, but to only a minority (<30 per cent) of the nodular sclerosing-type tumours.[120] These figures were subsequently confirmed in larger surveys of Hodgkin Lymphoma in the Western world, giving overall rates of EBV-positive disease in the 30–35 per cent range. By contrast, in Africa and less developed parts of South America where mixed cellularity-type disease was predominant, more than 90 per cent of Hodgkin tumours were EBV-positive. Other populations showed overall virus association rates between these two extremes.

Ironically, the hunt for a disease-associated virus had first been inspired by the unusual peak of tumour incidence in young adults in Western countries, but the nodular sclerosing-type tumours that were characteristic of this peak proved to have the lowest EBV-association. Initially this seemed at odds with the epidemiological evidence suggesting that young adults who acquired EBV late and developed infectious mononucleosis were immediately at increased risk of Hodgkin Lymphoma. That paradox was specifically addressed by epidemiologists at the State Serum Laboratory in Denmark. In an important study, they found that infectious mononucleosis was indeed associated with increased Hodgkin Lymphoma risk but that this was specific to the EBV-positive form of the tumour.[121] In fact, EBV-positive disease incidence was 20-fold higher between 2 and 3 years after infectious mononucleosis and only returned to base-line levels after 10 years, total EBV-positive case numbers during that decade being 4-fold more than expected. However, such post-infectious mononucleosis cases formed just a small fraction of the total young adult peak and so had little impact on the low overall EBV-positive rate seen among tumours in this age group. Exactly why the EBV-negative form of the disease occurs at such high incidence among young adults in the developed world remains a mystery to this day. Some still hold to the idea that late exposure to a yet-unidentified infectious agent could be involved, but so far no such agent has come to light.

What can we conclude from this complex intertwining of the Hodgkin Lymphoma story with that of EBV? Clearly this tumour can arise by at least two different routes, only one of which involves the virus. EBV-negative disease tends to present with a nodular sclerosing-type of cell infiltrate and accounts for most of the high incidence cases appearing in young adults in the West. By contrast, EBV-positive disease more often presents with a mixed cellularity-type of infiltrate and accounts for most cases of the disease seen in young children and older adults in the West, as well as for most cases of the disease seen in all age groups in less developed countries. However, these are trends rather than firm distinctions. In consequence, neither tumour type nor the age or nationality of the patient can be used as a reliable predictor of EBV's involvement. Both EBV-dependent and EBV-independent routes to malignancy culminate in the Reed-Sternberg cell, and their journeys to that destination probably involve at least some common steps.

Thus, all Reed-Sternberg cells began life as B lymphocytes and have the genetic signature of cells that have experienced antigen stimulation. That is, at some point they have entered into a phase of clonal growth and immunoglobulin gene mutation, just as happens to all antigen-stimulated B lymphocytes. However, unlike normal B lymphocytes which are programmed to die if they make inappropriate mutations, the cell that eventually turns into a Reed-Sternberg cell somehow escapes the death programme, thereby setting itself on the way to malignancy. In the case of EBV-positive tumours, the viral proteins LMP1 and LMP2 provide the escape route, activating cell survival pathways that signal life rather than death. In the parallel case of EBV-negative tumours, we now know that at least some have picked up rare mutations in the cellular genome that cause uncontrolled activation of those same survival pathways. What EBV can achieve in some circumstances, rare cellular mutations can achieve in others. In both cases, the result is the survival of a rogue cell that subsequently undergoes yet more mutations which not only promote growth but obliterate all other traces of its origin as a B lymphocyte. Finally we have it, the enigmatic Reed-Sternberg cell.

Most EBV-positive Hodgkin Lymphomas occurring later in life must arise as a long-term consequence of virus infection, that is, in individuals who are not obviously immune compromised and who have been carrying the virus asymptomatically for many years. Its appearance in those circumstances distinguishes Hodgkin Lymphoma from the EBV-associated Burkitt and post-transplant tumours, and invites comparison with another EBV-positive malignancy that develops in apparently immunocompetent virus carriers, nasopharyngeal carcinoma (NPC). Interestingly, these two tumours also share some other common features. First, when looked at under the microscope, both Hodgkin Lymphoma and NPC have an unusually large non-malignant cell infiltrate. In both cases many of the infiltrating cells seem to be attracted into the area by signals produced by the malignant cells themselves, as if much of the infiltrate were being induced to help tumour growth. Second, the two tumours share similar patterns of viral antigen expression involving EBNA1 and the LMPs, and in consequence remain potentially recognizable by the virus-specific T lymphocyte response. As described earlier, the most influential genes affecting NPC risk in Chinese people lie within the histocompatability (HLA) gene complex, and this HLA connection may relate to the individual's ability to mount a T lymphocyte response to EBV. Intriguingly, the same appears to be true of Hodgkin Lymphoma, at least in studies to date on Caucasian populations. Thus, in 2005, Poppema and colleagues discovered a link between genetic markers close to the HLA-A gene and susceptibility to EBV-positive, but not EBV-negative, disease.[122] Further work has now confirmed that HLA-A gene identity really is the factor that determines disease risk,[123] again implying an influence of T lymphocyte responses on tumour incidence.

Many questions still remain as to how the disease evolves, but the evidence for an EBV connection is now incontrovertible. Hodgkin Lymphoma represents a third type of EBV-associated B lymphocyte malignancy. For years this third association had been considered fanciful at best, not least because EBV was thought to be a virus of B lymphocytes, and the molecular evidence proving the tumour's B lymphocyte origin was still some way off. Then there was the surprising epidemiology of the EBV association: if a viral link existed at all, it was expected to be with the young adult form of the disease rather than with the form seen in young children and older adults. Not for the first time, EBV was defying expectations. And there was more to come.

* * *

The mantra that EBV infected B lymphocytes but not any other lymphoid cell types had held sway for more than 20 years. Then two reports published within a few months of each other in 1988, and an avalanche of reports that followed, changed everything. EBV was indeed finding its way into other lymphoid cells, and with dire consequences. In 1988 Jim Jones had just moved from Arizona, US, to set up a research group at the National Jewish Centre for Immunology and Respiratory Medicine in Denver. As a pediatrician, he had become interested in very rare patients, usually young children, presenting with a history of recurrent fevers, lymph gland enlargement, and malaise often lasting several years. The suspicion was that these chronic, infectious mononucleosis-like, symptoms were due to EBV infection, a suspicion that was reinforced by these patients' huge serum antibody responses to the virus, with levels reaching up to 100-fold greater than normal. Indeed, the presence of such very high level antibodies in serum, combined with a prolonged history of recurrent fever and lymph gland enlargement allowed clinicians to identify patients with a genuine 'chronic active EBV infection'. Importantly, such strict criteria also distinguished genuine cases of the chronic active condition from the hotchpotch of other chronic fatigue syndromes (sometimes called ME, myalgic encephalomyelitis) to which, in the 1980s, EBV was briefly and wrongly assigned as the causative agent. Impressed by the predictive power of EBV serology, Jones began to screen any patient with suggestive symptoms for high EBV antibody levels, hoping to find yet more EBV disease connections that, he believed, must be out there waiting to be discovered. As he now admits, somewhat self-effacingly, 'I was relatively new to the field and, at the time, probably thought that any disease with an infection and haematological/immunological components was likely due to EBV.' However wild such an assertion might seem, his instincts proved spectacularly correct.

Among the patients with high antibody titres were three individuals with T cell lymphomas. This was quite unexpected because all the available evidence argued against the possibility of any link between EBV and T cell tumours. Undeterred, Jones and colleagues checked the tumour samples from these three patients for viral and cellular markers. As they had dared to hope, the three tumours were indeed EBV genome-positive, even though each was derived from the CD4 subset of T lymphocytes. These results, published early in 1988, were the first evidence of EBV infecting any type of T lymphocyte, let alone being involved in a T cell lymphoma.[124] As Jones recalls, 'I guess that it was only my relative naivety in the field allowed me to ask questions about the virus being in T lymphocytes, particularly T lymphoma cells'—questions that others would probably have considered too far-fetched to bother with.

At the same time, and half a world away in Hokkaido University, Japan, another pediatrician, Hideaki Kikuta, was working with the country's leading EBV researcher, Toyora Osato. They had become interested in a rare inflammatory illness of children called Kawasaki disease, which some initial studies had suggested might be linked to primary EBV infection. To their dismay, all these early findings had come to nothing. They were left with a confusing set of results that Kikuta now recalls as 'being very difficult for me to explain, even in the Japanese language, let alone English!'. Little did they know how their fortunes were about to change. In 1987, a 2-year-old boy came to hospital with a five-month history of spiking fevers and enlarged lymph glands. He did not have typical symptoms of

Kawasaki disease but was nevertheless included in the study for interest. Serology quickly showed that this boy had undergone a recent EBV infection and that his virus capsid and early antibody levels had then risen to unprecedented heights, quite unlike anything seen in Kawasaki patients. Thinking that this might be an unusually severe case of infectious mononucleosis, Kikuta and colleagues looked in the blood expecting to see the picture characteristic of that disease, with some EBV-infected B lymphocytes and large numbers of CD8-positive 'killer' T lymphocytes. What they found was something completely different. The blood was full of activated CD4-positive T lymphocytes. This was surprising in itself, but even more surprising were the results of EBNA-staining. These activated CD4 T lymphocytes were not reacting against the virus infection: they themselves were EBV-infected and EBNA-positive. The virus had somehow tricked its way into T lymphocytes, the very cells that were designed to control it.

Kikuta's findings[125] were published in *Nature* in June 1988, just three months after Jones' report had appeared in the *New England Journal of Medicine*. Neither researcher knew of the other's existence; nor could they have imagined how their coincident findings would be forever interwoven in the history of EBV research. One study had focused on a Japanese child with a Kawasaki-like disease, the other on unusual cases of T cell lymphoma in the US. Yet closer inspection showed that they were not so far apart. The Japanese boy with Kawasaki-like disease looked very much like a classic case of chronic active EBV infection, while at least one of the three lymphoma patients in the US had developed their tumour within five years of suffering a severe primary EBV infection as an infant. Perhaps the two studies were looking at different ends of a single disease spectrum. The immediate effect of these findings was to break the conceptual stranglehold previously imposed by EBV's reputation as a virus exclusively infecting B lymphocytes and no other lymphoid cells. If the virus could occasionally infect CD4 T lymphocytes, perhaps it might also enter other white blood cell types, maybe even causing disease. New possibilities arose that would have seemed absurd just one year earlier, and some of those possibilities turned out to be true.

Though genuine cases of chronic active EBV infection were very rare, estimated to affect 1 or 2 children per million worldwide, they were somewhat more common in Japan, where all major centres had patients of this type. In the wake of Kikuta's findings, pediatricians working in Osaka looked at some of their patients and were struck by the fact that the blood picture was more often dominated, not by T lymphocytes, but by so-called 'granular lymphocytes'. These were in fact the natural killer (NK) cells that we have already met in earlier chapters, cells that work alongside T lymphocytes as part of the body's immune defence against an incoming virus. When the patients with NK cell proliferations were now studied, in many cases these NK cells were found to be EBV-positive[126] That led to further studies by several groups, in Japan and Taiwan in particular, focusing on children with chronic active or other symptomatic EBV infections. It turned out that in such patients sometimes CD4 T lymphocytes were infected, sometimes CD8 T lymphocytes, but most often this involved NK cells. The course of disease was also quite variable. In some cases T lymphocyte or NK cell infections could be rapidly fatal, with dramatic bone marrow failure. In other cases they produced the classical picture of chronic active EBV infection, with symptoms that could be stable for years but sometimes progressed into a T or NK cell lymphoma, with a single EBV-infected clone becoming fully malignant. Clearly, as one of the patients in Jones' 1988 report had hinted, chronic active EBV infection of the T (and NK) cells was a disease of ongoing cell proliferation, with a high risk of progression to full malignancy.

At this point, a picture was emerging of a variety of acute or chronic infectious conditions, all caused by EBV, but with malignancy on the margins as a rare long-term outcome. However a final piece of the jigsaw was still to be added, and this would put an EBV-associated cancer back at the centre of attention. Once again, the key observation came from Osato's research group in Hokkaido, Japan. They had extended their studies to include another syndrome which, though very rare in the West, was again more prevalent in Japan. This was a rapidly fatal disease of adults, usually presenting with erosion of bones in the nasal cavity and called lethal mid-line granuloma. In a curious parallel with the history of Hodgkin Lymphoma, this condition had been known since the nineteenth century, but for almost 100 years had been mistakenly considered a disease of uncontrolled inflammation rather than a malignancy. Then, in the early 1980s, researchers in Japan had shown it to be a lymphoma, probably of T lymphocyte origin. The possibility of a link to EBV seemed remote. However Osato and colleagues were intrigued by an earlier note in the *New England Journal of Medicine*, coming from clinicians in Paris and describing a patient with lethal mid-line granuloma who had IgA antibody responses to EBV rivalling those seen in NPC patients. Sure enough, Osato found that serum antibodies against the virus were very high in each of the first five Japanese patients tested. And then came the clinching evidence. All five cases of lethal mid-line granuloma were in reality EBV DNA-positive lymphomas and, by staining, the tumour cells were EBNA-positive. Based on cellular markers, two of these tumours were derived from CD4 T lymphocytes, while the others were almost certainly NK cell tumours.

These findings were published in *The Lancet* in 1990.[127] Though trailing Jones' original report by two years, this study was equally important since it provided the first evidence of EBV being consistently linked to a specific type of T or NK cell lymphoma. That link has since been reproduced in many other studies and, remarkably, every case of this rare disease examined worldwide proved to be EBV-positive. The consistency of this association, independent of geography, is strikingly similar to that shown by another tumour arising in the nasal cavity, NPC, and the pattern of virus gene expression in the two tumours is also similar. Perhaps most interesting is the higher incidence of this lymphoma, indeed of all the diseases associated with T/NK infection, in people of East Asian origin. This too is reminiscent of NPC, but there are important differences of detail suggesting that different susceptibility genes are involved. Thus NPC is most prevalent in South East Asia, particularly in people of southern Chinese origin, but is much rarer in the more northerly populations of northern China, Korea, and Japan. By contrast EBV-associated diseases of T/NK cell origin appear to be prevalent in all these Asian populations, with incidence rates much higher than in Caucasian populations of Europe and North America. Interestingly, in the Americas, cases of EBV-associated T/NK cell disease are most often seen in the indigenous population of Central and South America. These are people of East Asian origin whose ancestors appear to have carried their T/NK disease susceptibility with them in their migrations across the Bering Straits from Mongolia to Alaska, more than 10,000 years ago.

The causes and consequences of EBV straying from its usual B lymphocyte niche into the T lymphocyte and NK cells remain fascinating aspects of research to this day. Many of the questions that were first posed in the wake of the reports described above still have resonance. In the laboratory, the virus very efficiently infects B lymphocytes but, as yet, cannot be tricked into entering either T lymphocytes or NK cells. So we still do not know how the virus gets into these cell types in the body, how often that happens, or how latent EBV infection induces these target cells into growth and towards malignant change. It is sobering to think that the dangers of EBV's illicit entry into T and NK lymphocytes were first realized more than two decades ago, yet the secrets of EBV's life in these cell types remain largely unsolved. It's a timely reminder that, in science, one can never tell which questions will be easy to solve, and which will be frustratingly hard.

8

Prevention and Cure

Finding a cure for any type of cancer is a tall order but nevertheless by the mid 1960s it was apparent that Burkitt Lymphoma was an exception. As we saw in chapter 1, Denis Burkitt found that just one or two doses of cyclophosphamide, methotrexate, or vincristin generally caused even the largest tumours to shrink within a few days (see Figure 15). At the time cancer chemotherapy was in its infancy, so this rapid, sustained response was almost unprecedented, and for it to happen in Africa where cancer therapy was not a major priority seemed almost unbelievable. Ted Williams recalled an international conference on lymphoma in Kampala in 1965 where: 'Denis had gathered together all of his long-term survivors. When the delegates left the conference room for a tea break the children were outside, wandering around for the delegates to see: a bottle of Pepsi in one hand; and in the other photographs of themselves showing the tumour before chemotherapy was started.'[128] The delegates' response was complete incredulity.

While Burkitt was experimenting with chemotherapy in Kampala, Peter Clifford and Herbert Oettgen were also trying to find the best treatment for Burkitt Lymphoma in Nairobi. However, whereas Burkitt's policy was to induce a remission with as few drugs and as short a course as possible, sometimes using just a single dose, the other team were intent on using an intensive chemotherapy regimen designed to kill every last tumour cell in the body.

Burkitt's regime was clearly practical in the setting of Mulago hospital where the turnover time for patients in the children's ward was just 24 to 48 hours and parents often took children home as soon as their condition began to improve. However, once a child left hospital follow-up was difficult and the final outcome was often not known. So although Burkitt undoubtedly 'cured' a proportion of his patients, he could not confidently define the actual long-term survival rate.

Epidemiologists at Makerere University Medical School did their best to rectify this situation by tracing 55 of Burkitt's patients treated with chemotherapy between 1961 and 1965. By plotting a survival curve for these cases (Figure 16), the researchers illustrated an initial steep fall representing those that died during the treatment or had succumbed to a relapse shortly afterwards. This was followed by a more gradual decline in survival indicative of late,

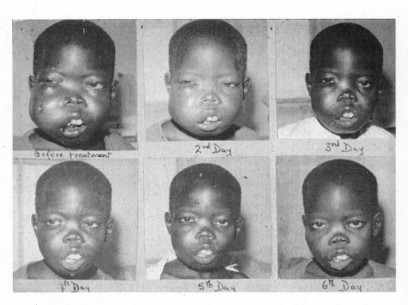

FIGURE 15 Photograph of a child with Burkitt Lymphoma shown before and 2–6 days after treatment with cyclophosphamide

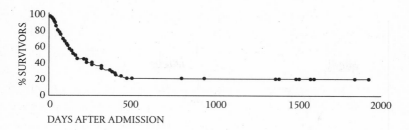

FIGURE 16 Chart showing the survival curve for Burkitt Lymphoma patients treated by Burkitt and colleagues.

fatal relapse. But then came the success story. What they describe as a 'striking, long, right-hand tail' (Figure 16), represented the survivors. Overall this included 11 of the 55 patients, giving a long-term remission rate of 21 per cent.[129] And although the report carefully avoids using the word 'cured', it does state that 'all of them have been clinically free from disease for at least 496 days, while the longest remission in a patient who has subsequently died is 382 days'. The same survival analysis on Clifford's treated cases using his more intensive chemotherapy regimen gave essentially similar results.[130]

Intriguingly, Burkitt occasionally witnessed spontaneous remission of tumours without any treatment, an event that never occurred with other types of lymphoma. Additionally, Clifford had seen cases with several late tumour recurrences, each of which he expected to be fatal but which responded completely to chemotherapy. Citing the case of one such small boy: 'He was in complete remission for almost a year after an initial dose of cyclophosphamide. Since then he has had: (1) a testicular tumour; (2) a bilateral submandibular tumour; (3) a recurrence of his original retroperitoneal tumour; (4) lymphoblastic meningitis; and (5) a tumour in the right cerebral hemisphere', all of which were successfully treated.[131] In the light of these observations both Burkitt and Clifford suggested that the immune response against Burkitt Lymphoma tumour cells must be an important factor in improving the final outcome of the treatment.

Clearly a more scientific approach was required to maximize the effect of chemotherapy and to investigate these potentially favourable immune responses. Fortunately help was soon at hand.

As we know, Burkitt's initial successes with chemotherapy attracted the interest of American doctors and this led to collaboration with chemotherapy experts from the US National Cancer Institute. As a result the 'Lymphoma Treatment Centre' opened at Mulago hospital in 1967 and John Ziegler, then a young doctor at the National Cancer Institute, became its first director. He arrived in Kampala in 1967 within months of Burkitt leaving for the UK.

Ziegler spent two years getting the centre up and running and touring the country's government and mission hospitals to encourage staff to refer Burkitt Lymphoma cases to the centre. By 1969 the centre, now re-named the Uganda Cancer Institute, had 40 research beds available for patients enrolled in cancer treatment trials, and Ziegler and colleagues began to address the pressing problem of how best to treat Burkitt Lymphoma. Since the lymphoma is such a fast-growing tumour, they knew that time was of the essence. The diagnosis must be made and treatment started within 24 to 48 hours of hospital admission to have the best chance of success. Sometimes the first line of treatment was surgical removal, or de-bulking, of the tumour. Although this was initially performed to relieve pressure on vital organs, it was later shown to hasten remission and be beneficial to long-term survival. The team identified several priorities, the first being to devise a clinical staging for the disease. As with any tumour this is based on the extent of the disease at presentation, with stage A (or in the case of nasopharyngeal carcinoma, stage I) being tumour localized to one site, and D (or IV) being widespread disease. This enabled different treatments to be given for the various stages, and separate outcomes to be monitored.

Another priority was to implement consistent observation and documentation of the clinical course of all patients. They insisted on frequent and long-term follow-up on every case, often a difficult call in tropical Africa but essential for accurately assessing the outcome of the treatment trials. Once these fundamentals were in place, the team was ready to carry out clinical trials comparing one drug combination with another, often giving more intensive therapy for late-stage disease. Like Burkitt, Ziegler and colleagues found that they could induce complete remissions with as little as one or two doses of cyclophosphamide. This was even so for patients with widespread disease, but, as Ziegler recalls: 'Not surprisingly, patients with a large tumour burden quickly relapsed after a single dose, so we used six doses as the "gold standard"'.

During the six years from 1967 to 1973 Ziegler and his team treated 192 Burkitt Lymphoma patients at the Institute. The survival curve for these patients was exactly the same *shape* as that produced by the epidemiologists at Makerere University for Burkitt's patients with its *striking, long, right hand tail*. But in this instance the tail was shifted in a very significant way. Overall, it now showed 50 per cent of patients were surviving,[132] and when plotted for stage A and B disease alone it contained a massive 73 per cent of cases. With their careful follow-up of these long-term survivors the researchers were now confident to say that they were cured—so how was this remarkable result achieved?

Overall, 157 of the 192 patients went into complete remission. Of the 157, full follow-up data were available on 141. By 1977–78, 69 of the 141 patients had died while 72 were alive and had been disease-free for between 4 and 10 years. The team found that tumour recurrence was rare after complete remission lasting for more than a year. However, they identified three separate high-risk time periods at which several deaths occurred that might be preventable: first, during treatment, second, within 3 months of treatment (early relapse), and third, between 3 and 12 months after treatment (late relapse).

Taking these risky periods in order, in the early trials around 10 per cent of patients died during treatment. These deaths were most common in children with very large, rapidly growing tumours. If these tumours did not respond immediately to chemotherapy they could kill by obstructing or destroying vital organs such as the airways or ureters. Another lethal, treatment-related complication was the 'acute tumour-lysis syndrome', first described by Ziegler and colleagues in relation to American Burkitt Lymphoma,[133] and later also found to occur during chemotherapy for other types of cancer. The syndrome results from a severe metabolic upset in patients with large tumours and poor kidney and/or liver function. Ironically, this is caused by the drugs doing exactly what they are designed to do—destroying large numbers of tumour cells. Unfortunately though, this releases masses of cell debris into the bloodstream. With normal liver and kidney function, the ion imbalance this causes can easily be handled, but in those with impaired function there is a danger of fatal cardiac arrest. Careful clinical and laboratory monitoring was required to prevent such a catastrophe.

Differentiating between early and late tumour relapse was key to a better understanding of the tumour response to chemotherapy since their causes and long-term prospects were quite different. Early relapse generally involved a recurrence at the site of the original tumour. This usually denoted resistance to the initial drug treatment and had a poor prognosis. In contrast, late relapses characteristically arose at a new site, often involving the central nervous system. This may have been caused by a few tumour cells surviving in organs where the drugs did not penetrate well. Alternatively, it could represent outgrowth of a completely new malignant clone. Surprisingly, late relapses responded well to chemotherapy and had a relatively good prognosis. As noted by Clifford, some children had several late relapses, all of which occurred within a year of each other. This sometimes continued for several years after the initial tumour, with each relapse often responding well to further chemotherapy. In this study a massive 43 per cent of long-term survivors had suffered relapses, some on up to six separate occasions—a most extraordinary statistic for relapsed cancer. Perhaps even more remarkable was the fact that tumour deposits in the brain were curable. Indeed the study figures show that 22 of the 72 long-term survivors had previously had a tumour in the central nervous system.

Interestingly, these unusual features of African Burkitt Lymphoma—high cure rates after multiple relapses and/or brain involvement—were not found in the rare cases of Burkitt Lymphoma in the US and Europe. These sporadic cases also required more intensive chemotherapy to induce a remission. To this day no one knows why two tumours of the same type should behave so differently, but at the time it was again suggested that the immune response to EBV in the virus-related, African tumours played a part in inducing remission. Consequently in one of the Ugandan studies, Ziegler and colleagues sought to stimulate the immune system and enhance any tumour-, or EBV-specific, responses. They knew that Burkitt Lymphoma patients had high levels of antibodies to certain EBV proteins and that the levels of anti early antigen and anti membrane antigen seemed to be of prognostic significance. Based on this knowledge, the team decided to administer BCG, the vaccine against tuberculosis, as a non-specific immune stimulant, and a vaccine prepared from X-irradiated cells from the patient's own tumour as a specific stimulant. They gave this concoction to patients who had achieved a complete remission on just two doses of cyclophosphamide in the hope that it might prevent tumour relapse. Unfortunately though, no such benefit was seen. The issue of whether the immune response is involved in Burkitt Lymphoma's rapid response to chemotherapy remains unresolved, but there is no doubt that the favourable outcome is at least in part due to the rapid growth rate of tumours before treatment. Anti-cancer drugs target growing cells and Burkitt Lymphoma is the fastest growing human tumour known. So with almost all the cells dividing every 24 to 48 hours, and an inbuilt instruction for programmed cell death if growth is interrupted (see chapter 4) it is no wonder that the tumours appear to melt away.

Ziegler returned to the US National Cancer Institute in 1972 and there followed a long, difficult period at the Institute in Kampala with unrest and civil war, the expulsion of Ugandan Asians, and mysterious disappearances among the staff. This continued until 1988 when peace was finally restored.

These early studies on the treatment of Burkitt Lymphoma had far-reaching consequences for tumour therapy in general and served as a model for the treatment of other lymphomas and leukaemias. While there are still problems relating to cost, drug availability, and patient compliance in the rural, tropical African setting, in the words of Ziegler: 'It is to the great credit of modern biomedical science that the many investigative implications of an unusual tumor discovered in a remote area of the world were so rapidly and effectively pursued'.[134]

* * *

Treatment for nasopharyngeal carcinoma, NPC, the second tumour to be discovered that is linked to EBV, is quite different from that of Burkitt Lymphoma. While first-line treatment for Burkitt Lymphoma is chemotherapy, for NPC it is radiotherapy. The treatment was pioneered by John Ho, whose contribution to NPC research and ideas on lifestyle-associated risk factors are described in chapter 5. Ho was a medical graduate from the University of Hong Kong who undertook post-graduate training in radiotherapy in the UK. He returned to Hong Kong in the early 1950s where he set up clinical radiotherapy services and a research laboratory from scratch and pioneered their use in the treatment of NPC. Ho was a dedicated clinician as well as researcher and he worked hard to improve the lot of NPC patients until his retirement in 1985. He was well aware of the many problems associated with the diagnosis and treatment of NPC. In particular, NPC, unlike Burkitt Lymphoma, does not present an obvious clinical picture. In its early stages the tumour is confined to a small primary growth in the nasopharynx. At this point (stages I and II disease) prompt treatment with radiotherapy gives around 90 per cent five-year survival. But unfortunately, localized disease is often either completely asymptomatic or produces a slight nasal discharge that is generally ignored. As a result, many patients only seek medical help after their tumour has begun to spread, typically presenting with swollen lymph glands in the neck with or without distant metastases.

This situation was improved in the mid 1970s when the blood test for IgA antibodies to the viral capsid antigen was shown to identify the small fraction of the population who were at particularly high risk of NPC (see chapter 5). This screening test was quickly adopted as a public-health measure in Hong Kong and several centres of high NPC incidence in China, so allowing cases to be picked up and treated at an early stage. Then in 1998 researchers in Thailand made another breakthrough. They were searching for cancer DNA markers in the blood of patients and since they knew that every NPC cell contained EBV, they reasoned that fragments of EBV DNA might be released from dying tumour cells and be detectable in blood plasma. Indeed this turned out to be the case,[135] and subsequently a group in Hong Kong optimized a new, highly sensitive test for detecting EBV DNA in plasma and clearly established its significance in relation to NPC. They found that 97 per cent of patients with the tumour were plasma-positive for EBV DNA compared with only 7 per cent of healthy controls. So not only was the assay sensitive, it was as specific as the IgA antibody assay and also technically much easier and quicker to perform.[136] Furthermore, like the IgA levels, EBV DNA levels in plasma correlated with tumour load but were much more rapidly responsive to changes in that load. Thus they could be used to monitor response to treatment—when patients with early-stage NPC were successfully treated with radiotherapy, levels of EBV DNA in plasma quickly rose to a sharp peak, coincident with the brief period of tumour cell killing, and then rapidly disappeared. Conversely patients who failed to respond never lost EBV DNA. Additionally, those who initially responded but then suffered a recurrence often became plasma EBV-DNA-positive again before the recurrence was visible on a scan.

While these technological advances did a lot to improve the outlook for NPC patients in high-risk areas, more precise tumour imaging and intensive radiotherapy have also played their part in improving overall survival rates. However, disseminated disease still presents a difficult clinical problem. At this stage intensive radiotherapy combined with chemotherapy is the treatment of choice, but although this may achieve a tumour response it is generally short lived and the prognosis is poor, with a median survival of 12 to 20 months.

* * *

Like NPC, the best treatment for early stage, localized Hodgkin Lymphoma is radiotherapy, which gives a cure rate of around 90 per cent. And again, for more widespread, late stage, or relapsing disease, intensive radiotherapy is combined with chemotherapy (sometimes accompanied by a stem cell transplant). Here the response rate is around 50 per cent but relapses occur and are difficult to treat. With these conventional treatments response rates for EBV-related and non-EBV-related Hodgkin Lymphoma are the same.

Clearly there is a continuing need to develop more effective therapies against all EBV-postive malignancies. In this regard, one of the most interesting new approaches is to use the human immune response as a basis for treatment. This takes advantage of the fact that all EBV-positive tumour cells contain virus-coded antigens, in other words proteins that should be recognised as foreign by the immune response. If immune cells making responses to these particular antigens did really exist, then they might be able to recognise and even destroy the tumour. But how would one find such cells in the vast army of cells making up the immune system? As it happened, they were uncovered by a pure stroke of luck.

* * *

In the late 1970s one of us, Alan Rickinson, then a lecturer in Anthony Epstein's department at the University of Bristol, took a sabbatical year to work in John Pope's laboratory at the Queensland Institute for Medical Research in Brisbane, Australia. This was the home town of Rickinson's wife, Barbara, and so it gave the chance both to visit family and work with another well-known EBV research group. It was here that Rickinson met Denis Moss, working in Pope's laboratory at the time, and the two began to work together. Both were interested in the biological mechanisms underlying EBV transformation of B lymphocytes, and previously each had used the cord blood system first described by Pope as well as Henle and Diehl in the late 1960s (see chapter 3). But in Brisbane it had become difficult to get cord blood so Moss and colleagues switched to using laboratory staff as voluntary blood donors. Now Rickinson began to infect blood lymphocytes prepared from adult donors for the first time, but was disappointed to find that many of the experiments failed. Clumps of infected B lymphocytes started to grow in the usual way for the first week or two, but then they dissolved and no cell lines grew out. Disappointment turned to curiosity, however, when he learnt that Moss and colleagues had also noted this early death of adult lymphocyte cultures in their recent work[137] but had never identified its cause. Intrigued, the two scientists set out to investigate the phenomenon that they called 'regression'.[138] Hopes were raised when they noticed that cultures containing lymphocytes from two EBV-seropositive laboratory workers showed regression while those from two EBV negative donors did not. But then EBV-infected lymphocytes from another donor, whose serum was regularly used as a negative control in EBV antibody assays, showed the strongest regression they had ever seen. At this point Rickinson admits that he asked himself: 'Is this all a wild goose chase?'

The answer to this question turned out to be a resounding no. When they rechecked the EBV antibody status of the strong regressor they got a real surprise. He had become EBV positive. Presumably he had experienced a silent primary EBV infection sometime in the previous few months. So regression appeared to be restricted to cells from people with a prior history of EBV infection after all—to quote Moss: 'The switch from cord blood to adult donor blood had unexpected rewards; now we knew we were onto something.'

In fact their culture system replicated what seems to happen inside the bodies of almost everyone who has been infected by EBV and then carries the virus for life—control of the infection by EBV-specific immune surveillance. In their experiments, the blood cell cultures comprised both B and T lymphocytes. When EBV was added to the mix it infected the B lymphocytes, inducing them to express the eight EBV latent proteins and begin to grow. While in the cultures from EBV-seronegative donors these infected cells grew out uninhibited, in the cultures from EBV-seropositive donors the viral protein-expressing B lymphocytes were recognized by pre-existing EBV-specific T lymphocytes and were promptly killed off.

Moss and Rickinson's studies were going on not long after two immunologists in Australia, Peter Doherty and Rolf Zinkernagel, had published experiments that would subsequently win them a Nobel Prize for Physiology or Medicine in 1996. They had found that, in mice, virus-specific T lymphocytes only recognized infected target cells if they were infected with the right virus and, crucially, if they expressed the correct "self" tissue type—that is the mouse equivalent of HLA antigens. This finding would have profound implications for the whole of immunology but, at the time, it was not clear whether the same rules also applied in humans. In one last, rushed set of experiments before Rickinson headed home to the UK, he and Moss took T lymphocytes from regressing cultures and added them to EBV transformed cell lines derived from people with the same and different HLA types. They found that the T lymphocytes only stopped the growth of cell lines that shared their HLA antigens, and not lines with unrelated HLA types. This was the first hint that the T lymphocytes causing regression were both virus-specific and HLA-restricted, as later studies would confirm. When Moss spent the year 1980–1981 in Bristol, the pair worked out how to grow these EBV-specific, killer T cells in culture, opening a way forward for them and many others to study the cell-mediated immune response to EBV, a feat that took many years.

One scientist who joined them in Bristol at this time was Cliona Rooney. Already in her mind was the possibility that these killer T cells might be useful as a way of treating EBV-positive tumours. After all, if such cells could recognize and kill EBV-transformed B lymphocytes in the laboratory, might they do the same to virus-positive tumour cells in the body? As a first step, she began to test these same killer T cells on EBV-positive Burkitt Lymphoma cell lines. The result was intriguing. The Burkitt Lymphoma cells were not recognized, even when they shared the same HLA type as the killer cells. This was the first clue that EBV in the Burkitt tumour was less visible to the immune response than it was in EBV-transformed normal B lymphocytes. The reason for this soon became clear. It turned out, as described in Chapter 6, that the virus was only making a single protein in Burkitt cells, EBNA1, and this was a poor target for killer T cells. Obviously, the goal of T cell therapy for all EBV-associated tumours was not going to be as easy as first thought. So where to begin? The answer was the tumour whose protein expression most closely resembled EBV-transformed B lymphocytes in the laboratory, post-transplant lymphoma.

By the early 1990s Rooney and her husband Malcolm Brenner, a haematologist and bone marrow transplantation expert, had moved to the US to work at St Jude's Hospital, Memphis, Tennessee. St Jude's is a charity-funded children's cancer hospital with a difference. Here research and treatment go hand in hand, so that every patient enters a clinical trial at the same time as receiving the best treatment free of charge. While Brenner set up a cutting-edge bone marrow transplant unit, Rooney was experimenting with T cell immunotherapy for those of his patients unfortunate enough to develop post-transplant lymphoma. Until this point in time the outlook for patients with post-transplant lymphoma was poor as they did not respond well to conventional chemotherapy or radiotherapy.

Brenner's transplant unit specialized in treating children with acute leukaemia, many of whom did not have an HLA-matched donor to provide the bone marrow they so desperately needed. In these cases it is common practice to use bone marrow cells from partially HLA-matched donors. But, this risks the T lymphocytes in the donor bone marrow attacking and killing the partially HLA-unrelated cells of the recipient. To circumvent this potentially fatal complication, doctors often remove the T lymphocytes from the donor marrow before infusion. But this procedure leaves the marrow recipients with very poor T cell-mediated immunity to control viruses, including EBV, a situation that lasts for up to a year. Thus, recipients of T lymphocyte-depleted marrows are at risk of uncontrolled growth of EBV-infected cells. Indeed, St Jude's records showed that in the past over 10 per cent of children transplanted with a partially HLA-matched, T-lymphocyte-depleted marrow developed post-transplant lymphoma.

Clearly this situation needed urgent attention and Rooney took up the challenge. Knowing that post-transplant lymphomas are almost all EBV-related and that the tumour cells express all eight EBV latent proteins, she argued that the tumours should be susceptible to EBV-specific killer T cells. Therefore, logically, she reasoned that replacing the patients' immune defect by infusing EBV-specific T lymphocytes derived from the bone marrow donor would provide a safe and effective way of preventing and/ or treating the disease.[139]

Rooney and colleagues carried out a series of clinical trials the first of which looked at the safety and efficacy of the proposed procedure. They grew EBV-specific T lymphocytes from healthy bone marrow donors and infused them into the bone marrow recipients. They then monitored the life span of the infused cells in the new host, their effect on blood EBV DNA load, and any adverse clinical reactions. The procedure involved growing literally hundreds of millions of EBV-specific T lymphocytes from the blood of each of 10 bone marrow donors in the laboratory, tagging the cells with a genetic marker so that they could be traced after infusion, and having them ready and waiting in the freezer by the time the transplant took place.

Each of the 10 recipients received an infusion of donor T lymphocytes between three and six months after their transplant. There were no toxic effects and the gene-marked lymphocytes remained detectable in the recipients' blood for an average of 10 weeks. Three of the 10 patients had high blood EBV DNA loads before the T lymphocyte infusion, an indication of uncontrolled growth of EBV infected cells, and indeed one of them was diagnosed with post-transplant lymphoma. In all three cases EBV DNA levels dropped dramatically after the infusions and the lymphoma resolved completely. These remarkable results allowed Rooney and colleagues to conclude that the infusions were safe and effective in controlling persistent EBV infection. They later used laboratory grown, EBV-specific T lymphocytes to successfully treat several patients with post-transplant lymphomas. Longer term follow-up showed that the infusions established a population of virus-specific killer T cells in the recipient that lasted for up to 18 months—long enough for the patient's natural immune function to be fully restored.[140]

The success of these trials established an important point of principle—that cell-based immunotherapy could be a credible alternative to radiotherapy and chemotherapy for treating cancer. Of course the model of post-transplant lymphoma in bone marrow recipients was an ideal starting point in every way—the tumours express viral proteins that are known targets for killer T cells, the bone marrow donors were available to provide T lymphocytes for growth in culture, following transplant the recipient's immune system was HLA identical to that of the donor, and the immune deficit that had allowed tumour growth was temporary.

Report of these trials heralded a whole new phase in clinical research into treatments for EBV-associated diseases and spawned several more clinical trials. In particular, there was a need for similar immunotherapy for post-transplant lymphoma following transplant of solid organs, now a credible treatment for terminally diseased kidneys, liver, heart, lungs, and small bowel. In this situation, described in chapter 6, the chance of lymphoma development is directly related to the amount of immunosuppressive drugs required to prevent rejection of the transplanted organ. Most at risk are those with heart, lung, and bowel transplants during the first year post transplant when levels of immune suppression are high. But as the drugs usually have to be continued for life, tumours may occur at any time. Also, primary EBV infection in immune suppressed people can lead directly to lymphoma outgrowth, and so those who are EBV negative before transplant, usually children, are at high risk. Indeed, the incidence of lymphoma in children's bowel transplant units can be as high as 20 per cent.

Not surprisingly, once Rooney's reports were published, the demand for killer T cells was overwhelming. But in most clinical situations production of these cells is just not practical. It takes around three months to grow enough cells to treat one patient. Since tumour patients cannot wait that long for treatment and no one can predict who will develop post-transplant lymphoma beforehand, ideally each high-risk patient undergoing transplant should have the cells ready and waiting in case they are needed. However, providing tailor-made cells for each patient is prohibitively expensive, labour intensive, and time consuming. Furthermore, with the exception of bone marrow transplants, organ donors are generally not alive or are not suitable lymphocyte donors.

For all these reasons Dorothy Crawford, now at the University of Edinburgh, UK, and her colleagues established a frozen bank of 100 EBV-specific killer T cells covering all the common UK HLA types. This could provide the required cells within days of a request. In the year 2000 the team began a multicentre clinical trial using the best HLA-matched killer T cells from the bank to treat patients with EBV-positive lymphomas, most being post-transplant lymphomas. This treatment was not without risk as infusions of killer T cells that were only partially HLA-matched to the recipient's HLA type could potentially damage recipient tissues. However, the team argued that as the killer T cells had been grown in the laboratory until they were entirely EBV specific they would only target EBV-infected cells. Fortunately, this turned out to be the case, and their dramatic effect is well illustrated by one particular case. This was not a transplant recipient but a young girl from Manchester, UK, with a congenital immunodeficiency. She had suffered from severe infections all her life and aged 8 she had a primary EBV infection followed by outgrowth of several EBV-positive lymphoma deposits in the brain. Every possible treatment was tried but all failed to control the tumours. Over a three-week period she went from being perfectly well to being unconscious on a ventilator in an intensive care unit. Only then did her doctors hear about the trial and contact the centre in Edinburgh. She was given several infusions of killer T cells from the bank and made a full recovery. Four months later she received a bone marrow transplant that corrected her immunodeficiency and has since led a normal, healthy life.[141]

Overall, 54 per cent of trial patients responded to treatment with the banked killer T cells and long-term follow-up showed no recurrences among the group that achieved complete remission.[142] Interestingly, around the same time another immunotherapy trial on post-transplant lymphoma was under way using the monoclonal antibody, rituximab. This antibody targets a protein called CD20 that is expressed on the surface of all B lymphocytes, including the EBV-transformed cells of post-transplant lymphoma, thus binding to, and killing, them. The trial reported a 40 per cent response rate— similar to the killer T cell therapy—although the antibody had no beneficial effect on tumours in the brain.[143] Obviously, giving injections of an off-the-shelf product like rituximab is much easier and cheaper than growing, storing, and administering live killer T cells even if they have been banked beforehand. Nevertheless, research aimed at refining cell-based immunotherapy for EBV-associated cancers continues in the hope of finding the ideal solution—perhaps a combined regimen including both antibody and cell-mediated arms of the immune response.

In recent years several groups have been attempting to extend this approach and use killer T cell preparations to treat NPC, relapsed Hodgkin Lymphoma, and T/NK cell lymphoma. The work is still at an early stage and has so far met with mixed results. This is likely due to the more restricted range of proteins present in these tumour cells typically involving only the EBNA1, LMP1, and LMP2 proteins, none of which are amongst the stronger targets for killer T cells. Nevertheless T lymphocytes directed against these particular proteins have now been detected in healthy, EBV positive people, and these can be cloned and grown up in the laboratory. This opens up the possibility of attacking the tumour cells with exactly the right type of killer T cell. In addition, scientists are trying to stimulate the patient's own immune response to these same proteins by vaccination. Such 'therapeutic vaccines' are specially designed so that, once they enter the body, they make harmless versions of those same EBV proteins so as to stimulate the patient's immune system to kill any cell expressing these foreign proteins.

* * *

The approaches discussed above all aim to improve the treatments available for EBV-associated disease once it has developed. But, increasingly, the ambition now is to develop a vaccine that can prevent EBV infection altogether, in other words a 'prophylactic vaccine' which would render people immune to infection before they are naturally exposed to the virus. Consider the benefits this would bring: EBV causes an estimated 250,000 cases of infectious mononucleosis and approximately 200,000 cancers annually worldwide (see Table 1), a disease burden that is clearly worth preventing. One of the major contributors to this total is NPC, but, rather surprisingly, the greatest single contribution to the global burden of EBV-associated tumours is estimated to be cancer of the stomach. As discussed in chapter 5, EBV is present in just a small minority of these tumours (2–10 per cent depending on the survey) but, because stomach cancer is so common on a worldwide scale, with nearly a million cases diagnosed annually, those containing EBV become hugely significant with regard to prevention.

The vaccine project was first suggested as a long-term goal by Epstein some 40 years ago. Initially, several hurdles were foreseen that had to be overcome. These included: (1) creating a vaccine that completely prevents infection, so-called 'sterile immunity', when the normal immune response to the virus does not prevent it establishing a life-long infection; (2) finding a suitable animal model in which to test candidate vaccines; and, (3) given the oncogenic nature of EBV, designing a vaccine that is safe to administer to humans. In addition, further down the line, the issue of when to give the proposed

TABLE 1 Estimated new cases of EBV-associated cancers worldwide per year

Cancer	Number of cases	Number of cases attributable to EBV
Burkitt lymphoma:		
Sporadic	400	100
Endemic	7800	6600
Gastric carcinoma	933,900	84,050
Hodgkin lymphoma	62,400	28,600
NPC	80,000	78,100
Total		197,450

From Cohen et al., Science Translational Medicine 3(107): 1–3. 2011. Reprinted with permission from AAAS.

vaccine has been much debated, because in most cases natural EBV infection occurs very early in life, yet vaccinating newborn babies does not generally induce a satisfactory immune response.

Epstein had always argued that preventing EBV infection would remove an essential link in the chain that leads to disease and thus an effective vaccine could prevent all EBV-associated disorders. At that time the cotton top tamarin was the animal model of choice for EBV lymphoma development, and so he set up a breeding colony at Bristol University with a view to testing candidate vaccines. A component of EBV membrane antigen complex called gp340/350 was known to induce antibodies that blocked EBV infection of B lymphocytes in the laboratory so this seemed the best vaccine candidate.

In 1985 Epstein and colleagues reported on experiments in which they successfully induced antibodies against gp340/350 in tamarins by immunizing with either a crude cell membrane preparation made from an EBV-transformed cell line expressing gp340/350 or with a purified form of the protein.[144] They challenged these animals with a dose of EBV known to cause tumours in 100 per cent of animals. In laboratory tests only serum from animals with high blood levels of gp340/350 antibody blocked EBV infection of B lymphocytes, and following EBV challenge, these were the animals that were protected from tumour development. The animals with lower levels of antibody and control non-immunized animals rapidly developed multiple, large tumour deposits. The team concluded that gp340/350 was a good EBV vaccine candidate that warranted further study. They knew that gp340/350 purified from an EBV-transformed cell line would not be deemed safe for use in humans. But after the entire EBV genome was sequenced in 1984 the gene coding for gp340/350 was revealed, and so the group suggested that this could be used to construct a safe, recombinant vaccine.

The pharmaceutical company GlaxoSmithKline was the first to try this out with the stated aim of preventing infectious mononucleosis. In 2007, company scientists reported on a clinical trial using a recombinant EBV gp340/350 subunit vaccine. The trial was randomized, double-blind, and placebo controlled, meaning that the 181 healthy, EBV negative student volunteers were randomly assigned to receive either the vaccine or a placebo. Neither the participants nor the trial organizers knew which formulation volunteers had been given until the code was broken at the end of the study. Ninety-nine per cent of the vaccinees produced antibodies to gp340/350 which remained detectable during the 18 months of the study. By the end, eight of the placebo group had developed infectious mononucleosis compared to just two of the vaccinees. This suggested some degree of protection but, during the 18 months, 9 of the placebo and 11 of the vaccinated group experienced silent primary EBV infection.[145] So although vaccination with gp340/350 appeared to reduce the symptoms of primary EBV infection it did not prevent the infection itself. Thus, for the time being, the dream of inducing sterile immunity was over. At least some virus particles has evaded gp340/350 antibodies to infect B lymphocytes. Furthermore, just one infected cell is probably enough to establish a persistent infection. Within a day or two this infected cell could proliferate into a whole clone of EBV-carrying cells, their growth only being controlled when the T lymphocyte response is established some 10 days later. So it was back to the drawing board for those interested in developing a vaccine to prevent EBV infection and disease.

Meanwhile, other scientists were taking a different approach to vaccine development. Encouraged by the success of killer T cell therapy at preventing and treating post-transplant lymphomas, they were looking at stimulating a T lymphocyte response against EBV proteins as a way of preventing EBV disease. While conceding that this strategy would not induce sterile immunity because killer T cells only recognze EBV proteins expressed by an infected cell, they thought that it would perhaps control the persistent infection at a low level and thereby prevent disease. In a small clinical trial Moss and colleagues administered a short sequence (a peptide) from the EBNA 3 protein known to be targeted by killer T cells expressing the HLA B8 antigen. Nine EBV negative, HLA B8 positive, healthy volunteers were inoculated, while four received a placebo.[146] The EBNA 3 peptide induced a specific T lymphocyte response in eight of the nine vaccinated volunteers, while none of the placebo group responded. But there is still a long way to go before this approach is feasible on a larger scale. The main drawback is the HLA restriction of T lymphocyte responses. For widespread application, scientists must find a way of incorporating peptides recognized by several HLA types into one vaccine.

The recent production and licensing of a vaccine to human papilloma viruses for preventing cervical cancer gave new impetus to the quest for a vaccine against EBV. In 2011 discussions got under way at the US National Institute of Health to find a way forward.[147] These deliberations endorsed gp340/350 as the best vaccine candidate while accepting that it may not be possible to induce sterile immunity. Nevertheless, the experts suggested that a vaccine that could control the level of persistent EBV infection had a good chance of preventing EBV disease. This hypothesis requires testing in a good animal model and here things have moved on since Epstein's tamarin experiments in the 1970s. It had been known for some time that Old World primates such as rhesus macaques were naturally infected with their own species of EBV-related herpesviruses. In the late 1990s scientists in the US took advantage of this to develop a potentially very important model. By careful hand-rearing animals from birth they established a colony of virus-free rhesus macaques and showed that these animals could be infected experimentally with the natural rhesus EBV-like virus.[148] Detailed analysis of the immune response to the rhesus virus is ongoing, but optimism is high that this virus infection in its natural host will prove a useful model for EBV vaccine development. Another advance is the development of the 'humanized mouse', which provides a much cheaper alternative to a primate model. The mice lack the genes necessary to develop their own immune system and so they can be transplanted at birth with human stem cells capable of reconstituting a normally functioning human immune system in the mice. This is still a rapidly developing research field, but it is already clear that delivering the virus to the human lymphoid tissues in these animals can reproduce at least some aspects of the EBV lifecycle in humans, with B lymphocyte infection and a corresponding T lymphocyte response.[149] The hope for the future is that this will provide a model in which the humanized mice can be given potential EBV vaccines and then challenged with the virus.

To date, experts are still divided on the best approach to producing an EBV vaccine and many questions remain—is preventing disease without preventing infection feasible? Will it be possible to design a single vaccine that prevents all EBV-associated diseases? Will a vaccine that stimulates both antibody and T lymphocyte arms of the immune response be required? We hope that between them the rhesus macaque and humanized mouse models will soon provide answers to these questions.

9

Making Sense of a Human Cancer Virus

We have been following the EBV story from the very beginning, ever since Anthony Epstein chanced to hear a talk by a little known surgeon, Denis Burkitt, about an unusual tumour of African children. The discovery of EBV in Burkitt Lymphoma marked the birth of a new field of investigation, that of human tumour virology, which has since grown to become one of the most important aspects of modern cancer research. How important we shall see later, with five more agents now known to be linked to human cancer and cases of virus-associated tumours accounting for more than 10 per cent of all cancers worldwide.[150] But first let us complete the EBV story and, in so doing, try to draw some important general conclusions. How can one virus contribute to so many forms of cancer yet, in most of us, be carried as a harmless infection? If we can understand that, then we will be reaching the goal of this final chapter: 'Making sense of a human cancer virus'.

As told so far, the story has read like an ongoing journey of discovery, the range of diseases linked to the virus increasing step by unexpected step. Every step along the way marked an area that then had to be explored in detail. Today these areas populate a landscape that encompasses the whole of EBV biology. At first glance, the landscape is dominated by the virus' many disease associations, the visible peaks of virus activity. But beneath those peaks are wide valleys where virus infection is taking its usual unremarkable course, present within the great majority of people but silent, never erupting into disease. We can appreciate this landscape from a distance, but we will never unlock its secrets until, as researchers, we walk in and explore things on the ground. To make sense of a cancer virus means to map its genes, to identify the proteins they encode, and to discover what those proteins do in the infected cell. That type of exploration needs years of laboratory work, often with research groups confined to particular parts of the landscape and studying the minutiae of molecular interactions therein. Literally thousands of people, far too many to mention, in groups all over the world have been explorers in this story. The picture we now have comes from them.

At the deepest level is the virus' genome, the genetic template that determines the virus' identity, its behaviour, its capacity to infect certain cells and not others, and ultimately its ability to cause disease. In chapter 6 we saw how, 20 years after EBV's discovery, the publication of its genome sequence[151] provided the tools that many laboratory scientists were looking for, opening the door to a detailed investigation of virus infection at the molecular level. In particular it led to identification of the eight latent proteins, six nuclear antigens (EBNAs), and two latent membrane proteins (LMPs), which underpin the virus' B lymphocyte growth-transforming ability. These proteins are made soon after the virus enters B lymphocytes and work together, first to activate the cells into growth and then to maintain those cells in the growth-transformed state. Understanding how the latent proteins act to disrupt cell growth control has been the focus of work in many laboratories for almost three decades. That work, running in parallel with the ongoing discovery of new EBV-associated diseases, has not only helped to make sense of those disease connections but has provided fascinating insights into the wider aspects of EBV's biology. Here we summarize some of the broad principles that have emerged.

The first of the EBNAs, EBNA1, has claims to be the most important latent protein, since it is present not just in B lymphocytes transformed in the laboratory but in every EBV-positive tumour. The reason for its ubiquity became clear when researchers in Wisconsin, US[152] found that EBNA1 is essential to prevent the EBV genome being lost from latently infected cells. The protein is physically bound to the viral DNA and ensures that, every time the cell divides, copies of that DNA are shared equally between the two daughter cells. EBV infections that involve proliferating cells, whether EBV-transformed cells in the laboratory or an EBV-positive tumour in the body, therefore depend upon EBNA1 to make sure that the infection is maintained. The other five EBNAs (2, 3A, 3B, 3C, and –LP) have different but equally important tasks, mainly concerned with activating cellular genes involved in cell growth. As first shown by groups in US and Germany using EBNA2 as the exemplar[153,154,155], these nuclear antigens work by physically piggy-backing onto particular cellular proteins that sit on the cell's DNA and control the activity of growth genes. That piggy-backing allows the individual EBNAs to multiply their effects, taking advantage of the many connections that the cell's own regulators of growth are programmed to make. Together, these EBNAs switch the cells growth-related genes permanently to the 'on' position.

The LMPs employ a similar trick, albeit working at the cell surface rather that in the nucleus. As shown by researchers in Harvard University, US[156,157], both LMPs act as mimics of particular cell membrane proteins that, in normal cells, receive growth and survival signals from outside and transmit those instructions to the cell nucleus where the responsive genes lie. The LMPs switch on the same signals and the cell responds, unaware that the instructions are coming, not from outside the cell, but from the virus within. The molecular details underpinning these activities are complex, but the guiding principle is worth restating. The virus has found a way of delving deep into the recesses of the cell and exploiting, for its own ends, pathways that are part of the cell's inbuilt programme of growth control. It does so by making viral proteins that, by clever molecular mimicry, can activate those pathways. The viral protein does not even need to look like the cellular protein in question, it just needs to carry a small region within its structure that mimics that protein and bind to the right partner within the cell. That binding is enough to generate a growth signal and the cell is programmed to obey.

* * *

Of course EBV has not acquired these proteins, or its ability to transform B lymphocyte growth, as some kind of malevolent strategy to cause disease. The transforming proteins have their place and are used at a particular point during the virus lifecycle in the body. But to understand this we have to take the long view and see that EBV is not unique in that regard: transforming ability is also a key property of viruses that are closely related to EBV and are found in our own closest evolutionary relatives, the Old World primates. Where studied, these viruses are shed through saliva and are carried for life as an asymptomatic infection of B lymphocytes, much as EBV is in humans. Furthermore, in the laboratory these EBV-like viruses are able to transform B lymphocytes of their own host species, and often of other primate species as well, using the same strategy as EBV itself. Kinship between these viruses is written in their DNA. EBV's Old World virus cousins have the same number of genes as EBV. These genes are arranged in the same order along the genome, and the genes themselves have similar sequences to their EBV counterparts. The closeness of the relationship between viruses is usually expressed as the degree of matching, termed 'homology', in the amino acid sequences of their proteins. One of EBV's cousins, the rhesus monkey virus already mentioned in chapter 8, has now been fully sequenced and its proteins were found, on average, to have a remarkable 75 per cent homology with those of EBV.[158] Interestingly, the latent proteins of the two viruses show slightly greater sequence differences, yet they still operate in much the same way, using similar tricks to achieve their ends.

This tells us that EBV and its Old World primate relatives have a common origin, just as do their Old World primate hosts. In each case the virus and its host species have been co-evolving in tandem for millions of years. Current estimates suggest that the two main lines of Old World primate evolution, one leading to the apes (including modern day humans) and the other to the monkeys, diverged some 25 to 30 million years ago. At that point of divergence, the last common ancestor must have carried its own ancestral virus from which EBV and all other EBV-like viruses of Old World primates are derived. From that time onwards, as the individual primate species developed their separate identities, so too the EBV-like viruses have co-evolved with their distinct hosts and acquired slightly different genomic sequences in the process.

How far back does this ancient virus-host interaction go? EBV-like viruses were thought to be restricted to Old World primates, because no antibodies cross-reacting with EBV had ever been seen in our next closest relatives, the New World primates of South America. Then, in the year 2000, scientists at the Regional Primate Center in Wisconsin were studying cases of spontaneous B cell lymphoma arising in their colony of common marmosets, a New World species, and found traces of herpesvirus-like DNA. Colleagues at Harvard University joined the hunt and, to their surprise, found a B lymphocyte-transforming virus that was a distant relative of EBV. The virus was soon fully sequenced,[159] with fascinating results. Compared to Old World viruses with their complement of over 80 genes, its genome is slightly smaller, with just over 70 genes, most of which are recognizable as being EBV-like even though the family resemblance is weak. In fact overall homology between the New World virus and EBV at the protein level is below 50 per cent, explaining why antibodies to one virus do not recognize the other. Once again, the greatest difference is in the latent proteins. Their number is reduced from eight to six in the New World virus, and the six that are present have diverged so far from their EBV counterparts that most can only be identified from the positions of their coding sequences on the virus genome. Yet, on close inspection, these New World virus latent proteins retain similar overall features, suggesting that they operate to transform B lymphocytes in much the same way as their Old World counterparts.

The discovery of an EBV-like agent in common marmosets was like a starting gun. Related viruses were soon being detected in other New World species, including spider and squirrel monkeys that had branched away from marmosets early in the course of South American primate evolution. Clearly EBV not only had close relatives among the Old World primates but a whole set of distant relations among New World primate species. What's more, both sets of viruses must have had a common origin, way back in evolutionary time. In that regard, all New World primates are thought to have evolved from ancestral species that migrated from the African land mass into the nascent continent of South America across an island trail or narrow land bridge some 30 to 50 million years ago, as the two continents split apart with the opening of the South Atlantic Ocean. Those New World founder species must have carried an EBV-like viruses with them, possibly not too dissimilar from the viruses present in New World primates today. Certainly, today's common marmoset virus gives a fascinating glimpse of what a primordial EBV-like virus might have looked like 50 million years ago. It probably had a slightly less complex gene set than today's EBV but it was already different from any herpesvirus ever seen before: it could infect and transform B lymphocytes.

* * *

To put this discovery into context, the herpesvirus family as a whole is divided into three sub-families called alpha (which includes human herpes simplex virus), beta- (which includes human cytomegalovirus) and gamma. The gamma sub-family is split into the EBV-like agents (called the gamma-1 viruses) and the human Kaposi sarcoma herpesvirus (KSHV)-like agents (the gamma 2-viruses). Viruses of the alpha-, beta- and gamma-2 type are found in host species across the animal kingdom, from primates to the mammals and, in some cases, in birds and amphibians. All these viruses replicate in one cell type in the body, producing infectious virus particles that can transmit the infection from one individual to another, and establish latency in another cell type, so that each infected individual carries the virus in silent form for life. For example, alpha-herpesviruses typically replicate in skin cells but go latent in neurons, cells of the nervous system. The EBV-like (gamma-1) viruses use an analogous strategy, in their case replicating in oral epithelial cells and going latent in B lymphocytes. However, they are distinct from all other herpesviruses in two important respects: they are restricted to primate hosts and they carry a unique set of growth-transforming genes specifically designed for use in latency.

Thus gamma-1 viruses represent the most recent branch of herpesvirus evolution, one that dates back a mere 100 million years and goes hand in hand with the evolution of the primates. Furthermore, their special ability to colonize primate B lymphocytes is beautifully reflected in their genes. First, gamma-1 viruses all have a unique gene, not seen in any other type of herpesvirus, encoding a protein (gp 340/350 in EBV) that lies on the outer face of the virus particle and binds specifically to a cellular protein on the B lymphocyte surface. This binding acts like a key opening a lock, providing the virus with very efficient entry into its preferred target cell. But gamma-1 virus specialism does not end there. The eight transforming genes themselves encode proteins that are uniquely adapted to work together in B lymphocytes. In addition, a further adaptation ensures that these eight genes can only be activated together in that type of cell. Strategically placed upstream of the transforming genes in the viral genome there are a series of control sequences that recruit the B lymphocyte's own gene-activating proteins, leading the cell itself to kick-start the virus' growth-transforming programme. The whole thing happens like clockwork because, over millions of years of evolution, the gamma-1 herpesviruses have honed an ability to make B lymphocytes their natural home and to exploit that particular cell's make-up for their own ends.

Evolution has endowed all herpesviruses with an ability to establish latency in a particular cell type in the body. With the exception of the gamma-1 viruses, this has been achieved without them acquiring a special set of growth-transforming latent genes. That begs the question as to what has driven evolution of the gamma-1 virus' unique growth transforming ability. Virus-transformed cells are clearly a potential threat to the life of the host, so what overriding advantage did the transforming genes bring to the ancestral gamma-1 herpesvirus? As with many questions in science, we do not know for certain. However, we can make an educated guess. Herpesviruses are highly successful agents that, over millennia, have diversified to infect many host species across the animal kingdom. Central to that success has been these agents' ability to establish lifelong latent infections.

Latency allows an individual host, infected in infancy, to carry the virus silently for years and then, much later, to reactivate the infection and pass infectious virus on to another individual. This capacity for periodic transmission frees the virus from dependence upon a continual supply of new, uninfected individuals to maintain its presence in the host population. In theory, just one successful transmission every host generation would be enough to guarantee the virus' survival. As a result, herpesvirus infections can be maintained in quite small host communities, for example in isolated founder populations from which new host species evolve. But the success of this strategy depends entirely upon latent infections being long lasting in the individual host, and this is best achieved if the type of cell harbouring that infection is itself long lived.

Viewed in this light, the ability of alpha-herpesviruses to establish latency in neurons gave them a key advantage, since cells of this type naturally survive for the lifetime of the host. By contrast, such an advantage is not given to the gamma-1 viruses, which have evolved to infect B lymphocytes. The majority of those cells have much shorter life spans. In fact, as we discuss below, the only B lymphocytes to survive long term are those that have been specially selected as 'memory cells', the few cells that happen to have made the best antibodies against any previous infection. Now we can begin to see the advantage that acquiring the transforming genes might have given EBV and its primate cousins. It allowed them to overcome the unpredictability of the B lymphocyte's lifespan. Transformation mimics the natural process of antigen exposure and memory selection, thereby guaranteeing that latently infected B lymphocytes gain the characteristics of memory cells.[160] The growth-transforming programme, written in the latent genes of every gamma-1 herpesvirus, allows the virus to create its own long-lived home.

* * *

That said, the gamma-1 virus lifestyle is not without its dangers. Growth-transforming ability generates cells that, if not controlled, will grow and kill the host. Indeed, had there been no control, the primordial transforming gamma-1 virus would have been expunged from the evolutionary record millions of years ago; it would literally have died out along with the few host individuals it managed to infect. Instead it survived and flourished because the primate immune system provided, not only the B lymphocyte niche to harbour latent infection, but also the T lymphocyte surveillance to keep that infection under control. It is only when that evolutionary balance is disturbed that disease ensues.

We saw this illustrated graphically in chapter 6 with transplant patients receiving immune suppressing drugs which impair T lymphocyte function. Such immune suppression breached an evolutionary contract that took virus and host millions of years to reach, and post transplant lymphoma, the uncontrolled outgrowth of virus-transformed B lymphocytes, was the predictable result. It is therefore not difficult to make sense of EBV's role as the cause of post-transplant lymphoma. By contrast, EBV's role in the development of other B lymphocyte tumours is more complex. Both the Burkitt and Hodgkin Lymphomas, are rare accidents occurring during the virus's normal life in B lymphocytes. Like most accidents, they are unpredictable and depend upon the coincidence of several untoward events. Some of these accidents are completely independent of the virus and stem from the uniquely dangerous lifestyle that B lymphocytes themselves display. As we have noted, the normal function of these cells within the immune system is to make antibodies against foreign antigens. Any one such antigen can only be recognized by a tiny fraction of the total B lymphocyte population, and it is on these few cells that an effective antibody response depends. To maximize that response, antigen-stimulated B lymphocytes are programmed to expand rapidly, producing many daughter cells that are copies of themselves. At that point, something happens that is quite unique: each daughter cell starts randomly mutating their immunoglobulin (antibody-coding) genes so that the daughter population as a whole contains many different variants of the original immunoglobulin sequence. Then the body will select only the few daughter cells whose variant immunoglobulin best fits the original antigen challenge, and will discard the rest. It is those highly selected cells, capable of making the most effective antibodies to the antigen in question, that are then kept and enter the long-lived 'memory' pool.

Now set this in the context of lymphoma development. There is a low but finite risk that such deliberate mutation of the immunoglobulin genes, will produce mistakes, genetic accidents predisposing to cancer. Indeed, such accidents do occasionally happen. This very probably explains why the great majority of all lymphomas seen in humans come from B lymphocytes and not from other types of lymphoid cell. More importantly, in the specific setting of Burkitt and Hodgkin Lymphomas, the risk of a cell carrying a genetic accident and then progressing to malignant lymphoma is greatly enhanced when the cell involved is also infected with EBV. In Burkitt Lymphoma, the chance chromosomal translocation leading to uncontrolled activation of a cellular oncogene, c-myc, is thought to occur as an accident of immunoglobulin gene mutation. Very rarely, this can combine with other cellular changes to produce the Burkitt tumour without any involvement of EBV. However, the presence of the virus alongside the translocation greatly increases the risk of malignant change. Similarly in Hodgkin Lymphoma, cellular genetic changes, likely to include accidents of immunoglobulin gene mutation, combine with EBV to produce the malignant Reed-Sternberg cell. Clearly it is possible to reach the same end-point without the virus' involvement, as is apparent from the young adult peak of Hodgkin Lymphoma in the Western world. But the young adult disease is actually the exception: most cases of the tumour worldwide are EBV-associated.

In both Burkitt and Hodgkin Lymphomas, EBV contributes to tumor cell growth and survival, not through classical growth trans-formation, but through more restricted forms of infection, involving just a subset of latent proteins. Again, these more restricted forms have not been devised for the malevolent purpose of causing disease: they are aspects of the virus' usual behaviour in the B lymphocytes it which it persists. Because B lymphocytes normally pass through various stages during their lifespan, the virus has evolved to behave accordingly at each stage, switching on only those viral genes necessary for the infected cell to survive. While it is difficult to catch virus-infected cells at those stages in healthy virus carriers, we see them amplified in the Burkitt and Hodgkin tumours. Forms of infection that are used fleetingly in the virus's normal life have been permanently captured in these tumours. Why? Because the viral genes being expressed are actively contributing to tumour development.

So much for the tumours of B lymphocyte origin; now let's turn to the virus-associated tumours of other cell types. Arguably, these are not accidents of the virus' normal lifestyle in the body but rare consequences of the virus infecting the wrong cell type. Such infec-tions are of no survival advantage to the virus: they are cul-de-sacs in which it can neither establish a useful persistence nor replicate to escape. Yet such infections are potentially dangerous because the virus finds itself in an environment where the normal rules no longer apply. Without the B lymphocyte signals to kick-start transformation, the virus falls back on alternative patterns of latent infection involving just a subset of vital genes. In T and NK lymphocytes, even this limited subset of virus latent proteins seems able to promote cell growth and to predispose the cells to future malignant change. In epithelial cells, the same proteins appear to act later in the disease process, as in the case of nasopharyngeal carcinoma (NPC) where EBV enters an already pre-malignant cell and moves it on towards malignancy. This may also be true of those cases of gastric carcinoma that carry the virus. There are even reports of the virus being found in rare epithelial tumours arising at certain other body sites[161] as well as in bizarre tumours derived from smooth muscle cells that arise in heavily immunocompromised patients, particularly HIV-infected children.[162] It would appear that EBV's oncogenic potential is no respecter of cell lineage: all it needs is the opportunity afforded by chance infection of the wrong cell type.

* * *

So where does EBV now stand in the pantheon of human tumour viruses, that elite group of agents of which it was the founding member and which has now grown to include at least five more virus types? Of these, it remains not only one of the most interesting but also the virus linked to the most diverse range of tumour types. The closest comparator turns out to be none other than EBV's nearest relative among the eight known human herpesviruses, the Kaposi sarcoma-associated herpesvirus (KSHV). This virus was discovered in 1994, exactly 30 years after the discovery of EBV, by two scientists working at Columbia University in New York, Yuan Chang and Patrick Moore.[163] Reminiscent of the Burkitt Lymphoma story, Chang and Moore found the virus through its association with a human tumour, Kaposi sarcoma, which mainly occurred in Africa, but in the 1980s had exploded to prominence as a high incidence tumour of immunocompromised AIDS patients. Since then, KSHV has been linked to all cases of Kaposi sarcoma worldwide, as well as to a rare B lymphocyte malignancy (pleural effusion lymphoma) that is almost exclusively seen in end-stage AIDS. The virus naturally infects endothelial cells, from which the sarcoma is derived, and a number of white blood cell types including B lymphocytes, which again are the main site of virus latency. But KSHV, a gamma-2 herpesvirus, lacks EBV's classical growth-transforming ability and establishes much lower levels of latent virus in B lymphocytes. Nevertheless, KSHV deservedly takes its place as the second human herpesvirus to be linked with cancer, a link that again involves more than one type of malignancy.

The other human tumour viruses come from different virus families. Best known are the human papilloma viruses, small DNA viruses whose association with cervical cancer and other epithelial tumours of the genital tract was first reported in 1974.[164] That discovery was made by Harald zur Hausen, the person whose long-standing interest in tumour viruses had been boosted by his early years working on EBV in the Henles' laboratory. Zur Hausen was awarded the Nobel Prize for his papilloma virus work in 2008, the year in which Chang and Moore made yet another addition to the list of human tumour viruses. This time it was a small DNA virus of the polyoma virus family, whose strong association with a rare form of skin cancer, Merkel cell carcinoma, is apparent from its assumed name, the Merkel cell virus.[165] Both papilloma and polyoma tumour viruses are quite widespread in human populations, usually as innocuous infections of epithelial cells. Occasionally, however, instead of replicating in the normal way in these cells, the viral DNA becomes accidentally integrated into the cellular genome. If that happens in such a way that the virus' growth-promoting proteins are permanently switched on, then the cell is driven into unscheduled growth and one step has been taken on the way to fully malignant change.

Two other types of human tumour virus are also thought to act by inserting copies of their genomes into cellular DNA. One of these, hepatitis B virus, does so as an accident of its chronic infection of liver cells and is linked to many cases of liver cancer worldwide.[166] Another, a retrovirus called human T lymphotropic virus (HTLV)1, integrates into the cellular genome as part of its normal replication cycle and is linked to a rare form of adult T cell leukaemia.[167] In both cases cancer occurs in only a small fraction of infected people, usually after many years of virus carriage and through the combined action of viral damage and cellular genetic change. The human tumour viruses are therefore surprisingly varied in type, yet they share similarities in terms of their association with malignant disease. Generally virus-associated cancers are rare accidents of persistent infection by a virus that is often widespread in the population and in most cases is carried asymptomatically. Moreover, the virus is typically one link in a complex chain of events leading to malignancy, but it is often the most recognizable link, and one that can tell us much about how and why cancer occurs.

* * *

This brings us up to date with the EBV story and places the virus in a wider contemporary context. From that perspective, let us briefly consider what lessons can be learned from the past 50 years of EBV research, not just about virus infections, but also about the scientists who study them and the nature of the scientific process itself. On the first point, the sheer diversity of diseases linked to EBV shows just how varied and how complex the biology of a virus can be. Here we have an agent that has co-evolved with our ancestral species for millions of years, taking an evolutionary course that might be viewed as high risk by infecting and establishing latency in B lymphocytes, acquiring the growth-transforming genes necessary to establish persistence in that cell type and also the flexibility to activate different combinations of these genes at different stages of that cell's life history. Such is the selective power of evolution that, by the time our immediate ancestors came down from the trees and walked upright on the African savannah, the EBV-host balance was firmly struck. The virus was able to persist and spread, in most cases without threatening the life of the individual host. Yet the potential for malignancy was always there, written in the virus' growth-transforming genes. Rare circumstances can allow that oncogenic potential to be realized but, because only a small fraction of the virus-carrying population ever develops a virus-associated tumour, in evolutionary terms such cases do not impact on the continued survival of both the virus and its host species.

Clearly, EBV is pathogenic, yet we cannot blame the virus for all associated diseases. There are circumstances where man himself intervenes, breaking the evolutionary contract between virus and host, and creating problems in the process. The case of post-transplant lymphoma has already been discussed, but this is not the only example of a recent man-made disease. An unintended consequence of the West's cultural change to a more hygienic lifestyle is that many individuals do not acquire EBV until the teenage years or later, at which time they are at risk of infectious mononucleosis. In effect this is a new disease which has arisen in affluent societies precisely because the natural cycle of early virus transmission has been broken. Why delayed, but not early, infection should predispose to infectious mononucleosis is not entirely understood. However, it may relate to the maturing of the human immune system over the first two decades of life, since the disease is now thought to be immune mediated. In other words, the symptoms of fever, lymph node enlargement, and fatigue are not caused by the virus infection per se but by an over-active T lymphocyte response to the infection. Infectious mononucleosis, like post-transplant lymphoma, is therefore 'caused' by EBV in the formal sense, but in both cases the circumstances allowing disease to arise are actually man-made.

What then of the scientists who have played their part in the EBV story? They are too many and varied to name in a book of this kind, and we must let their collective achievements speak for them. Save for Epstein, the Henles, and the Kleins who were the founding parents of EBV research, only a few individual names have escaped the editors' scythe. Some of those names will be familiar to present devotees of the virus, but others will not. That is the way of it in science. There are some like Harald zur Hausen who made deliberate and telling impacts on the EBV story before moving on to make an indelible mark in other fields. There are others whose equally important contributions were made unwittingly, chance findings that arose in the course of work begun for entirely different reasons and then left for others to explore. And there are those for whom the virus became something of a lifelong obsession, figures in a landscape in which they could always find an interesting, if not comfortable, niche.

Most important to record is the contribution that clinicians have made to the development of the field. Many new areas of EBV research, from Burkitt Lymphoma, through X-linked lymphoproliferative disease and post-transplant lymphoma to the diseases of T/NK cell infection, began when an odd patient caught an inquisitive clinician's eye. Sometimes those leads bore early fruit, as when Epstein began work on the tumour that Denis Burkitt first brought to the world's attention. But other leads were left unappreciated for several years. Why was it, for instance, that more than a decade elapsed between the first reports of lymphoma in kidney transplant patients in 1968/1969 and the first clear evidence of EBV's involvement published in 1980/1981? Partly it was the problem of access to samples from transplant centres where the disease presented erratically, often with patients only diagnosed in extremis. But partly it was because, with an abundance of existing disease connections to study, most EBV researchers were too engrossed in their own business to give post-transplant lymphoma the attention it deserved. That is why a research community needs to be a broad church, not just of different disciplines but of different temperaments. It needs both those who walk in and explore things on the ground and those who survey the landscape from on high, the doers and the dreamers if you like. All have their contribution to make.

Our story also tells us something about the practice of science itself. There are many vignettes showing just how unpredictable research can be, and how often serendipitous events are the key to progress. Epstein could not have foreseen how his impromptu attendance at Denis Burkitt's lecture on 22 March 1961 would change the course of his working life. His decision on that day, to drop everything and work on an unusual tumour of African children, was inspired yet also full of risk. The whole project might have floundered had not this lymphoma been one of very few human tumours that could be reproducibly grown in culture, had not the cell culture environment encouraged a few tumour cells to activate their latent virus and make virus particles, and had not Epstein been a trained electron microscopist and therefore able to see a virus that, at the time, was undetectable by any other virus test. Equally tenuous were the circumstances that in 1966 opened sceptical eyes to the possibility of a second EBV-associated malignancy, NPC. It just so happened that Peter Clifford, the ENT surgeon in Kenya sending Burkitt Lymphoma patients' sera to Herbert Oettgen and Lloyd Old in New York, by chance included sera from his NPC patients among the non-Burkitt controls. And was it circumstance or fate that Elaine Hutkin, a technician working in the Henles' laboratory and their favourite seronegative control, should contract infectious mononucleosis and come back to work EBV antibody-positive? These are but a few examples to make the essential point. Research does not always move along the logical lines that written reports seem to imply. It is essentially a journey without maps, where sudden insights light up the way ahead, only to reveal a number of possible onward trails, many of them false.

Yet eventually truth will out, one way or another. If the EBV story were to be re-run from scratch, we would very likely arrive today at a similar landscape but by a different route. Had Epstein never looked at Burkitt Lymphoma, the virus would eventually have been discovered, possibly in the spontaneously transformed cell lines that, even as early as 1963,[168] were emerging as unrecognized guests during attempts to grow human leukaemia cells in culture. Certainly it would have been found, very likely by electron microscopy, in the same cell lines that by 1967 were known to arise rapidly in lymphocyte cultures from infectious mononucleosis patients.[169] That would soon have led to the virus being identified as the cause of infectious mononucleosis, but its links to malignancies such as Burkitt's Lymphoma and NPC might have taken years to uncover. And the early history of human tumour virology would have been all the poorer as a result.

* * *

So much for history. What of the future? Where might the next 50 years take us? Predictions are notoriously difficult to make in science because research, by its very nature, so often takes an uncharted course. However, there are some intriguing questions to be addressed in the coming decade and, looking even further ahead, some important long-term goals.

Though the EBV genome sequence has long been known, we still do not understand the function of many of the virus' 80 or so genes. In the laboratory, as many as a third of these are not required either for the virus to transform B lymphocytes or for it to replicate and produce infectious particles. That does not mean these genes are redundant: they almost certainly play important roles in real life, but those roles are not detected in our limited laboratory models of virus infection. From the little that we do know about them, some of these genes probably help to prolong the life of infected cells in the body, while others assist the virus in avoiding elimination by the host immune response. Then there are other genes about which we know even less, including some that do not code for proteins at all but are simply transcribed as short RNAs that have important effects in their own right. Two of these, the so-called EBER RNAs, have been known for many years and are abundant in latently infected cells, but their functions remain enigmatic. Recently, these have been joined by another 30 or more small RNAs (known as micro-RNAs), each with their own unique sequence and each encoded by mini-genes hitherto unrecognized on the viral genome. These EBV-coded micro-RNAs are predicted to regulate the activity of many cellular genes, thereby providing the virus with a further layer of control though which to influence the behaviour of infected cells. Exactly which cellular genes are regulated in this way, and what the consequences are, remain to be seen. But the take-home message is clear: there is still a huge amount to learn about the full complement of EBV genes in the virus genome, about when and where they are active, and what those genes can do.

At the heart of things, there will always be the fascination with EBV as a tumour virus. We still need to understand in molecular terms the complex sequence of events that lead to EBV-positive tumours. Work continues apace on the behaviour of the virus in tumours but, with the exception of Burkitt Lymphoma, we still know little about the cellular genetic changes that act with the virus to produce malignancy. Yet, as the example of Burkitt Lymphoma shows, it is only when these cellular changes are identified that we can really begin to see what complementary role the virus plays. There are hopes of progress in this area now that the entire genome of cancer cells can be sequenced, and scientists can look for key genomic changes that are common to cancers of a certain type. Such work has already begun, with NPC being the first EBV-associated tumour in line. Cancer genome sequencing has enormous long-term potential, but right now we are in the phase of data-gathering and it is too early to say what the outcome will be. The objective is no less than a complete understanding of the route, or routes, whereby cancer develops.

Meanwhile, given the history of EBV's ever-expanding links to human cancer, can we now say that the list of EBV-associated malignancies is complete? The answer is 'probably yes', though it would be a brave soul who would state this categorically. There may still be very rare tumours of unanticipated cell types, like the EBV-positive smooth muscle cell tumours seen in HIV-infected children, which will continue to surprise. But almost all common tumours must by now have been screened for EBV infection without further additions to the list.

Perhaps more important for the future is to broaden the above question and ask, can we now say that the list of EBV-associated diseases is complete? This is more controversial, but the temptation is to answer 'probably no'. This is particularly true in the context of autoimmune diseases, conditions in which one or other body tissue is attacked by the patient's own immune cells. What could trick the immune system into attacking self in this way? A constant theme of research on such diseases is the possibility that the triggering event is some kind of viral infection, where the virus-induced immune response contains elements that by chance cross-react with self antigens present in particular tissues. In that regard, one of the most devastating of autoimmune diseases is multiple sclerosis, where immune attack leads to irreversible damage to the central nervous system. The incidence of this disease is influenced by several factors thought to impact on immune function,[170] but the question of the involvement of a virus has long been uppermost in researchers' minds. Many aspects of the disease epidemiology, particularly the high incidence rates seen among young adults in the developed Western world, are consistent with it being triggered by late acquisition of a common virus. Remarkably, the serological evidence now strongly suggests that, of all common viruses, the only agent whose acquisition increases disease risk is EBV.[171,172] In fact, EBV-carriers are 15-fold more likely to develop the disease than matched EBV-negative controls. Moreover, the lifetime risk of multiple sclerosis is increased a further two to three-fold in individuals with a history of infectious mononucleosis. Conceivably, the EBV-induced immune T lymphocyte response contains elements which, in rare circumstances or in rare individuals, can go on to cause the damage that underpins this progressive neurologic disease. It is important to say that this postulated link between EBV and multiple sclerosis is still highly controversial but, at the time of writing, the circumstantial evidence is becoming stronger. Here the lessons of history implore us to keep an open mind. Only time, and much further research, will resolve the issue. But the EBV–multiple sclerosis connection emphasizes how, even after 50 years of research on this extraordinary virus, entirely new areas of work continue to open up.

Let us finish with what is undoubtedly one of the most important long-term goals for the EBV research community. As we have seen, the virus is linked to an astounding array of different diseases and its impact on human health worldwide is indisputable. All this disease burden is potentially avoidable if we could prevent EBV infection altogether by vaccination. Though such a project faces many scientific and logistic hurdles, the call for an EBV vaccine becomes ever stronger. This will surely double in intensity if the recently forged link between the virus and multiple sclerosis holds true, particularly if, as with infectious mononucleosis, the risk of that disease were to be linked to late primary infection. One could then imagine a targeted vaccination programme focusing on children who were still EBV-negative as they entered the teenage years and were therefore at risk for infectious mononucleosis and, possibly, also multiple sclerosis. Likewise, vaccination to prevent the more common virus-associated malignancies would in the first instance have to be targeted, for example to infants born into families with a known history of NPC. This may sound ambitious but the concept of vaccination against a cancer-causing virus has become a reality in the past decade with the success of the human papilloma virus vaccine. That example shows what is possible, providing one has a vaccine that confers long-lasting immunity against infection. Unfortunately there are many differences in biology between human papilloma viruses and EBV, and studies to date suggest that the strategy underpinning papilloma vaccine design may not be sufficient to protect against a cancer-causing herpesvirus. Indeed there are doubts as to whether a vaccine fully protective against EBV infection can ever be achieved. Opinions are divided, and that is exactly why the work needs to be done. After all, science is about setting an important question and seeking to resolve it by reason and experiment, hopefully spiced with a little serendipity. What greater challenge could a new generation of EBV researchers ask for?

NOTES

INTRODUCTION

1. Medawar P and Medawar JS. *Aristotle to Zoos: A philosophical dictionary of biology.* Harvard University Press, Cambridge, Mass. US. 1983.

CHAPTER 1: OUT OF AFRICA

2. In B Glemser *The long safari.* Scientific book club. 1971, p25–6.
3. Epstein Sir A and Eastwood MA. Denis Parsons Burkitt. 28 February 1911–1993. Biographical memoirs of fellows of the Royal Society, 41: 90. 1995.
4. Epstein Sir A and Eastwood MA. Denis Parsons Burkitt. 28 February 1911–1993. Biographical memoirs of fellows of the Royal Society, 41: 90. 1995.
5. In B Glemser *The long safari.* Scientific book club. 1971, p42.
6. Burkitt DP. Cancer 51: 1777. 1983.
7. Burkitt DP. Cancer 51: 1777. 1983.
8. Burkitt DP. Cancer 5: 1778. 1983.
9. Burkitt DP. Br J Surg. 46: 218–23. 1958.
10. O'Conor GT and Davies JNP. J Pediat. 56: 526. 1960.
11. Wright DH. Brit J Cancer 17: 50. 1963.
12. Cooper EH et al. Europ J Cancer 2: 377–84. 1966.
13. Burkitt DP Cancer 51: 1779. 1983.
14. Burkitt DP Cancer 51: 1779. 1983.
15. Booth K et al. Brit J Cancer 31: 657–64. 1967.
16. Dalldorf G. et al. Perspectives in Biology and Medicine 7: 435–49. 1964.
17. Kafuko GW and Burkitt DP. Int J Cancer 6: 1–9. 1970.
18. Pike M et al. Brit J prev. soc. Med 24: 39–41. 1970.
19. Kafuko GW and Burkitt DP. Int J Cancer 6: 1–9. 1970.
20. Burkitt DP Cancer 51: 1784. 1983.

CHAPTER 2: THE EUREKA MOMENT

21. Rous P. J Exp Med. 13: 397–411. 1911.
22. Borrel A. Annals Inst. Pasteur 17: 81–122. 1903.
23. Ellermann V and Bang O. Zentralbl. Bakt. Abt. I (Orig). 46: 595–609. 1908.
24. Bittner JJ. Science 84: 162. 1936.
25. Epstein MA Nature 181: 1808. 1958.
26. Epstein MA and Barr YM. Lancet i: 252–3. 1964.
27. Epstein MA and Barr YM. J. US Nat. Cancer Inst. 34: 231–40. 1965.
28. Pulvertaft RJV. Lancet i: 252–3. 1964.

29. Epstein MA et al. J US Cancer Inst 37: 547–59. 1966.
30. Epstein MA, Achong BG, Barr YM. Lancet i: 702–3. 1964.
31. Epstein et al. J Exp Med.121: 761–70. 1965.

CHAPTER 3: CONVINCING THE SCEPTICS

32. Henle G and Henle W. J Bact 91: 1248–56. 1966.
33. Henle W et al. Science 157: 1064–5. 1967.
34. Pope JH et al. Int J Cancer 3: 857–66. 1968.
35. Jondal M and Klein G. J Exp Med 138: 1365–78. 1973.
36. Yefenof E et al. Int J Cancer 17: 693–700. 1976.
37. Dalldorf G. JAMA 181: 1026–8.
38. Evans AS. Am J Med Sci. 267: 189–95. 1974.
39. Hoagland RJ Am J Med Sci. 229: 262–72. 1955.
40. Pope Nature 216: 810–1. 1967.
41. Henle G et al. PNAS 95: 94–101. 1968.
42. Henle G et al PNAS 95: 94–101. 1968.
43. Chang RS and Golden HD.Nature 234: 359–60. 1971.
44. Henle G et al. J Nat Cancer Inst. 43: 1147–57. 1969.
45. Hallee JT et al. Yale Journal of Biology and Medicine 3: 182–95. 1974.
46. Sayer RN et al. J Infect Dis 122: 263–70. 1971.
47. University Health Physicians and PHLS. BMJ. 4: 643–6. 1971.
48. Balfour HH et al. J Infect Dis 207: 80–8. 2013.
49. Crawford et al. J Infect Dis. 186: 731–6. 2002.
50. Zur Hausen et al. Nature 228: 1056–8. 1970.

CHAPTER 4: EBV IN AFRICA

51. In *The Long Safari*. B Glemser, Scientific book club. 1971. p188.
52. In *The Long Safari*. B Glemser, Scientific book club. 1971. p190.
53. <www.iarc.fr/> (accessed 22 August 2013).
54. de-Thé et al. Nature 274: 756–61. 1978.
55. Pike MC and Williams EH. BMJ 2: 395–9. 1967.
56. de-Thé et al. Nature 274: 756–61. 1978.
57. Werner et al. JID 126: 678–81. 1972.
58. Epstein et al. Int J Cancer 12: 309–18. 1973.
59. Shope et al. PNAS 70: 2487–91. 1973.
60. Klein G and Klein E. Ann Rev Immunol. 7: 1–33. 1989.
61. Klein G and Klein E. Ann Rev Immunol. 7: 21. 1989.
62. Zur Hausen et al. Nature 228: 1056–8. 1970.
63. Adams A and Lindahl T. PNAS 72: 1477–81. 1975.
64. Pope JH et al. Nature 222: 186–7. 1969.
65. Rowe M et al. EMBO J. 6: 2743–51. 1987.

66. Manolov G and Manolova Y. Nature 237: 33–4. 1972.
67. Zech et al. Int J Cancer 17: 47–56. 1976.
68. Shimizu et al. J Virol 68: 6069–73. 1994.

CHAPTER 5: EBV IN ASIA: NASOPHARYNGEAL CARCINOMA

69. Old et al. PNAS 56: 1699–704. 1966.
70. zur Hausen et al. Nature 228: 1056–8. 1970.
71. Nonoyama et al. PNAS 70: 3625–8. 1973.
72. Wolf et al. Nature New Biol 244: 245–7. 1973.
73. Klein et al. PNAS 71: 4737–41. 1974.
74. Wara et al. Cancer 35: 1313–15. 1975.
75. Henle and Henle, Int J Cancer 17: 1–7. 1976.
76. Zeng et al. Int J Cancer 29: 139–41. 1982.
77. Zeng et al. Intervirology 20: 190–4. 1983.
78. Liu et al. Am J Epidemiol 177: 242–50. 2013.
79. Buell, Cancer Research 34: 1189–91. 1974.
80. Wee et al. Chinese J Cancer 29: 510–26. 2010.
81. Simons et al. Int J Cancer 13: 122–34. 1974.
82. RaabTraub and Flynn, Cell 47: 883–9. 1986.
83. Greenspan et al. N Engl J Med 313: 1564–71. 1985.
84. Lo and Huang, Semin Cancer Biol 12: 451–62. 2002.
85. Tsang et al. PNAS 109: E3473–82. 2012.
86. Shibata et al. Am J Pathol 139: 469–74. 1991.
87. Shibata and Weiss, Am J Pathol 140: 769–74. 1992.

CHAPTER 6: NEW EBV DISEASES: AN ACCIDENT
OF NATURE, AN ACCIDENT OF MEDICINE

88. Bar et al. NEJM 290: 363–7. 1974.
89. Purtilo et al. Lancet 1: 935–40. 1975.
90. Provisor et al. NEJM 293: 62–5. 1975.
91. Purtilo et al. Am J Med 73: 49–56. 1982.
92. Coffey et al. Nature Genetics 20: 129–35. 1998.
93. Nichols et al. PNAS 95: 13765–70. 1998.
94. Sayos et al. Nature 395: 462–9. 1998.
95. Sullivan et al. J Clin Invest 71: 1765–78. 1983.
96. Parolini et al. J Exp Med 192: 337–46. 2000.
97. Penn, Transplant Proc 7: 323–6. 1975.
98. Calne et al. Lancet 2: 1033–6. 1979.
99. Bieber et al. Lancet 1: 43. 1980.
100. Nagington and Gray, Lancet 1: 536–7. 1980.
101. Crawford et al. Lancet 1: 1355–6. 1980.

102. Hanto et al. Surgery 90: 204–13. 1981.
103. Fialkow et al. Lancet 1: 251–5. 1971.
104. Thomas et al. Lancet 1: 1310–13. 1972.
105. Schubach et al. Blood 60: 180–7. 1982.
106. Baer et al. Nature 310: 207–11. 1984.
107. Starzl et al. Lancet 1: 583–7. 1984.
108. Ziegler et al. NEJM 311: 565–70. 1984.

CHAPTER 7: UNEXPECTED ARRIVALS: HODGKIN LYMPHOMA AND THE T/NK CELL LYMPHOMAS

109. Hodgkin, Med Chir Trans 17: 69–97. 1832.
110. Sternberg Z Heilk 19: 21–91. 1898.
111. Reed, Am J Med Sci 124: 653–69. 1902.
112. Kuppers et al. PNAS 91: 10962–6. 1994.
113. Johansson et al. Int J Cancer 6: 450–62. 1970.
114. Rosdahl et al. BMJ 2: 253–6. 1974.
115. Connelly and Christine, Cancer Res 32: 1174–8. 1974.
116. Veltri et al. Cancer 51: 509–20. 1983.
117. Poppema et al. Am J Clin Pathol. 84: 385–90. 1985.
118. Weiss et al. Am J Path 129: 86–91. 1987.
119. Howe and Steitz, PNAS 83: 9006–10. 1986.
120. Pallesen et al. Lancet 337: 320–2. 1991.
121. Hjalgrim et al. NEJM 349: 1324–32. 2003.
122. Diepstra et al. Lancet 365: 2216–24. 2005.
123. Hjalgrim et al. PNAS 107: 6400–5. 2010.
124. Jones et al. NEJM 318: 733–41. 1988.
125. Kikuta et al. Nature 333: 455–7. 1988.
126. Kawa-Ha et al. J Clin Invest 84: 51–5. 1989.
127. Harabuchi et al. Lancet 335: 128–30. 1990.

CHAPTER 8: PREVENTION AND CURE

128. In B Glemser The long safari. Scientific book club. 1971, p136.
129. Morrow RH et al. BMJ 4: 323–7. 1967.
130. Pike MC Lancet ii: 856. 1966.
131. Pike MC Lancet ii: 856. 1966.
132. Ziegler JL et al. Lancet ii: 936–8. 1979.
133. Cohen LF et al. Am J Med. 68: 486–91. 1980.
134. Ziegler JL New Engl J Med. 305: 735–45. 1981.
135. Mutirangura et al. Clin Cancer Res 4: 665–9. 1998.
136. Lo et al. Cancer Res 59: 1188–91. 1999.
137. Moss DJ and Pope JH Int J Cancer 15: 503–11. 1975.

138. Moss DJ et al Int J Cancer 22: 662–8. 1978.
139. Rooney CM et al. Lancet 345: 9–13. 1995.
140. Heslop HE et al. Nature Med. 2: 551–5. 1996.
141. Wynn RF et al. Lancet Oncology 6: 344–6. 2005.
142. Haque T et al. Blood 110: 1123–31. 2007.
143. Choquet S et al. Blood 107: 3053–7. 2006.
144. Epstein MA et al. Nature 318: 287–9. 1985.
145. Sokal EM et al. J Infect Dis 196: 1749–53. 2007.
146. Elliott SL et al. J Virol 82: 1448–57. 2008.
147. Cohen JI et al Science transplantation medicine 3(107): 1–3. 2011.
148. Moghaddam A et al. Science 276: 2030–3. 1997.
149. Traggiai E et al. Science 304: 104–7. 2004.

CHAPTER 9: MAKING SENSE OF A HUMAN CANCER VIRUS

150. Pisani et al. Cancer Epidemiology, Biomarkers and Prevention 6: 387–400. 1997.
151. Baer et al. Nature 310: 207–11. 1984.
152. Yates et al. PNAS 81: 3806–10. 1984.
153. Ling et al. PNAS 90: 9237–41. 1993.
154. Grossman et al. PNAS 91: 7568–72. 1994.
155. Zimber-Strobl et al. EMBO J 13: 4973–82. 1994.
156. Mosialos et al. Cell 80: 389–99. 1995.
157. Longnecker et al. J. Virol. 65: 3681–92. 1991.
158. Rivailler et al. J. Virol. 76: 421–6. 2002.
159. Rivailler et al. J. Virol. 76: 12055–68. 2002.
160. Babcock et al. Immunity 9: 395–404. 1998.
161. Leyvraz et al. NEJM 312: 1296–9. 1985.
162. McClain et al. NEJM 332: 12–18. 1995.
163. Chang et al. Science 266: 1865–9. 1994.
164. zur Hausen et al. Int J Cancer 13: 650–6. 1974.
165. Feng et al. Science 319: 1096–100. 2008.
166. Beasley et al. Lancet 2: 1129–33. 1981.
167. Poiesz et al. PNAS 77: 7415–19. 1980.
168. Benyesh-Melnick et al. JNCI 31: 1311–31. 1963.
169. Pope, Nature 216: 810–11. 1967.
170. Ascherio et al. Nat Rev Neurol 8: 602–12. 2012.
171. Ascherio and Munger J Neuroimmune Pharmacol 5: 271–7. 2010.
172. Levin et al. Ann Neurol 67: 824–30. 2010.

FURTHER READING

CHAPTER 1

Magrath I. Brit J Haem. 156: 744–756. 2012.
Epidemiology: clues to the pathogenesis of Burkitt Lymphoma.
Glemser B. *The long safari*. Scientific book club. 1971.

CHAPTER 2

Epstein MA. Brit J Haematol. 156: 777–779. 2012.
Burkitt Lymphoma and the discovery of Epstein-Barr virus

CHAPTER 3

Williams H and Crawford DH. Blood 107: 862–869. 2006.
Epstein-Barr virus: the impact of scientific advances on clinical practice

CHAPTER 4

Grommonger S et al. Brit J Haematol. 156: 719–729. 2012.
Burkitt lymphoma: the role of Epstein-Barr virus revisited
Bornkamm GW. Semin Cancer Biol. 19: 351–365. 2009.
Epstein-Barr virus and its role in the pathogenesis of Burkitt's Lymphoma: an
    unresolved issue
Moormann AM, Snider CJ, Chelimo K. Curr Opin Infect Dis. 24: 435–441.
    2011.
The company malaria keeps: how co-infection with Epstein-Barr virus leads to
    endemic Burkitt Lymphoma

CHAPTER 5

Lung ML. Seminars in Cancer Biology 22(2): 77–78. 2012. (And articles therein)
Unlocking the Rosetta stone enigma for nasopharyngeal carcinoma: genetics,
    viral infection, and other environmental factors
Shah KM, Young LS. Clin Microbiol Infect. 15: 982–988. 2009.
Epstein-Barr virus and carcinogenesis: beyond Burkitt's Lymphoma
Iizasa H, Nanbo A, Nishikawa J, Jinushi M, Yoshiyama H. Viruses. 4: 3420–3439.
    2012.
Epstein-Barr Virus (EBV)-associated gastric carcinoma

CHAPTER 6

Rezaei N, Mahmoudi E, Aghamohammadi A, Das R, Nichols KE. Br J Haematol. 152: 13–30. 2011.
X-linked lymphoproliferative syndrome: a genetic condition typified by the triad of infection, immunodeficiency and lymphoma
Green M, Michaels MG. Am J Transplant. 13 Suppl 3: 41–54. 2013.
Epstein-Barr virus infection and posttransplant lymphoproliferative disorder

CHAPTER 7

Hjalgrim H. Dan Med J. 59: B4485. 2012.
On the aetiology of Hodgkin Lymphoma
Farrell K, Jarrett RF. Histopathology. 58: 15–25. 2011.
The molecular pathogenesis of Hodgkin Lymphoma
George LC, Rowe M, Fox CP. Curr Hematol Malig Rep. 7: 276–284. 2012.
Epstein-Barr virus and the pathogenesis of T and NK lymphoma: a mystery unsolved
Imashuku S. Pediatr Hematol Oncol. 24: 563–568. 2007.
Systemic type Epstein-Barr virus-related lymphoproliferative diseases in children and young adults: challenges for pediatric hemato-oncologists and infectious disease specialists

CHAPTER 8

Sandlung JT. Brit J Haematol. 156: 761–765. 2012.
Burkitt Lymphoma: staging and response evaluation
Zeigler JL. Brit J Haematol. 156: 766–769. 2012.
Into and out of Africa—taking over from Denis Burkitt
Bollard CM, Rooney CM, Heslop HE. Nat Rev Clin Oncol. 9: 510–519. 2012.
T-cell therapy in the treatment of post-transplant lymphoproliferative disease
Lee AW, Ng WT, Chan YH, Sze H, Chan C, Lam TH. Radiother Oncol. 104: 272–278. 2012.
The battle against nasopharyngeal cancer
Chan ATC. Annals of Oncology 21 (Suppl 7): vii308–vii312. 2010.
Nasopharyngeal carcinoma
Long HM et al. Curr Topics in Immunol. 23: 258–264. 2011.
Immune defence against EBV and EBV-associated disease

CHAPTER 9

Young LS, Rickinson AB. Nat Rev Cancer. 4: 757–768. 2004.
Epstein-Barr virus: 40 years on
Javier RT, Butel JS. Cancer Res. 68: 7693–7706. 2008.

The history of tumor virology
Owens GP, Bennett JL. Mult Scler. 18: 1204–1208. 2012.
Trigger, pathogen, or bystander: the complex nexus linking Epstein- Barr virus
and multiple sclerosis
Tselis A. Curr Opin Rheumatol. 24: 424–428. 2012.
Epstein-Barr virus cause of multiple sclerosis

GLOSSARY

Antibody: A generic name for a class of proteins called immunoglobulins (Ig)/ gamma-globulins that are found in blood and body fluids and are produced by B lymphocytes as part of the host's immune response to specific antigen. There are three main classes of antibody molecules, IgM, IgG, and IgA. IgM and IgG antibodies are made during a primary infection but, whereas IgM antibodies are transient, IgG antibodies are detectable in serum for many years. IgA antibodies tend to be made in response to infections of mucous membranes such as the lining of the lungs and gut. They can be detected locally in secretions and also in serum. Antibodies against particular antigens on the surface of microbes have the potential to render the microbes non-infectious, so called 'neutralizing antibodies'.

Antigen: A foreign substance, usually a protein, capable of inducing an immune response.

Atypical mononuclear cells: Large, activated, CD8 T lymphocytes found in blood during the early stages of acute infectious mononucleosis (glandular fever).

B cell/lymphocyte: A subset of lymphocytes that make antibodies during an immune response.

Capsid: Virus-encoded protein shell that protects the virus genetic material.

CD4 T cells/lymphocytes: A subset of T lymphocytes that express the CD4 molecule on their surface. Also called 'helper T cells' as they 'help' other lymphocyte subsets to generate the host's immune response.

CD8 T cells/lymphocytes: A subset of T lymphocytes that express the CD8 molecule on their surface. Also called 'killer T cells' because, once they recognize a cell infected with a specific virus, they can kill that cell.

Chromosomal translocation: The accidental transfer of part of one chromosome onto another, causing a genetic abnormality.

Chronic active EBV infection: A chronic disease with prolonged or recurrent infectious mononucleosis-like symptoms, caused by EBV and marked by very high antibody responses to the virus.

Chronic fatigue syndrome: A disabling fatigue of at least six months' duration that is not relieved by rest and occurs in the absence of recognizable predisposing conditions. Also called myalgic encephalomyelitis (ME). Despite earlier claims, this condition has no association with EBV.

DNA hybridization: A molecular biology technique that uses a complementary DNA probe to detect target DNA in a sample by binding (hybridizing) to it.

Early antigen: An antigen expressed in those EBV-infected cells that are in the early stages of virus production.

EBERS: Two EBV-encoded small RNAs that do not encode proteins. These RNAs are found in all latently infected cells, including EBV-positive tumours. Their function is still uncertain, but it is thought that they may play a role in tumour development.

EBV receptor: The CD21 molecule on the surface of B lymphocytes to which EBV binds prior to entry into the cell (see Gp340/350).

Endothelial cells: Cells that line the inner walls of blood vessels.

Gp340/350: A glycoprotein (gp) expressed by EBV as part of the membrane antigen complex. A specific interaction between this glycoprotein and the CD21 molecule on the B lymphocyte surface (see EBV receptor) allows EBV to infect B lymphocytes preferentially.

Growth transformation: The conversion of a normal cell into a continuously growing cell line. Experimental EBV infection of B lymphocytes in the laboratory causes their growth transformation. Spontaneous growth transformation may also occur in the laboratory when B lymphocytes from an EBV carrier are cultured without addition of the virus.

Histocompatibility leucocyte antigens (HLA): A complex of protein molecules (self antigens) on the surface of cells that determine a person's unique tissue type. There are two main classes of HLA antigens: class I antigens are present on virtually all body cells; class II antigens are expressed on lymphocytes and certain other cell types involved in the immune response. CD8 T lymphocytes have receptors that detect slight changes in HLA class I antigens, such as occur when a cell is infected with a virus. Infection with a particular virus activates only that small fraction of the body's CD8 T lymphocytes whose receptors specifically recognize HLA changes induced by that virus; those activated T lymphocytes become killer T cells and go on to destroy virus-infected cells. CD4 T lymphocytes have receptors that recognize slight changes in HLA class II antigens, such as occur when other cell types involved in the immune response take up viral proteins released from infected cells.

HLA restriction: This describes a basic rule that governs how T lymphocytes function. During their development in the body, T lymphocytes have been selected to recognize virus-induced changes occurring only in the context of self-HLA antigens. They cannot recognize changes in the HLA antigens of a different individual, even if those changes are induced by the same virus. As a result, T lymphocytes are said to exhibit 'self-restriction', usually referred to as 'HLA-restriction'.

Immunofluorescence staining: A laboratory technique used to visualize recognition of an antigen within individual cells by a specific antibody added from outside. Recognition produces an antigen–antibody complex, and that complex is visualized either directly (by having the antibody pre-labelled with a fluorescent tag) or indirectly (by adding a fluorescent-tagged third reagent that will bind to the antibody within the complex). Fluorescence staining is detected by examining the cells under a microscope and illuminating with ultra-violet light. Such staining can be used either (i) to detect the presence of a particular antigen within cells by using a pre-labelled antibody known to be specific for that antigen, or (ii) to detect the presence of any particular antibody reactivity within a serum sample by testing that serum on cells known to contain the relevant antigen, and visualizing any antigen–antibody complex formed using a pre-labelled third reagent.

Immunoglobulin genes: Genes that code for antibody molecules (immunoglobulins/gamma-glublins). In humans, the immunoglobulin heavy chain genes are on chromosome 14, and the immunoglobulin light chain genes are on chromosomes 2 and 22. These genes are active in antibody-producing B lymphocytes.

Immunosurveillance: The ability of immune cells, particularly T lymphocytes that have responded to a previous virus infection, then to patrol the body for life, seeking out reactivated or new infections with the same virus and controlling them.

In situ hybridization: A molecular method for specifically detecting genetic material, for example virus genome sequences, within individual cells in a specimen by binding (hybridization) with a specific probe complementary to the sequence in question.

Kaposi sarcoma: A virus-associated endothelial tumour named after the Hungarian dermatologist who first described it. Presents a slow-growing form in elderly men of Mediterranean, Eastern European, or Jewish origin, and clinically more aggressive forms in young Africa males and in immunocompromised individuals such as HIV-AIDS patients or immunosuppressed transplant recipients. Caused by Kaposi sarcoma herpesvirus, a human gamma-2 herpesvirus discovered in 1994.

Kawasaki disease: An autoimmune disease of endothelial cells (lining blood vessels) that occurs in early childhood and affects multiple organs. The most serious outcome is disease of the coronary arteries.

Killer T cells/lymphocytes: See T lymphocytes.

Lymphoepithelioma: An epithelial tumour that contains a large infiltration of non-malignant lymphocytes, hence the frequent use of this term to describe nasopharyngeal carcinoma.

Membrane antigen: An EBV antigen complex expressed on the surface of infected cells during virus replication and present on the virus envelope. It includes the receptor-binding protein gp340/350 that binds to B lymphocytes and mediates their infection.

Memory cells: Long-lived B and T lymphocytes that have responded to an antigen and retain the ability to respond again, thereby preventing or ameliorating illness on a second encounter with the same antigen. For both B and T lymphocytes, only a small fraction of cells involved in the first response to antigen are selected into memory. In the case of B lymphocytes, selection is reserved for those cells making antibodies that show the strongest recognition of the original antigen.

Micro-RNAs: Small non-coding RNA molecules that are naturally expressed in cells and are involved in regulation of cellular gene expression; EBV is one of several larger viruses that encode their own micro-RNAs.

Molecular mimicry: The concept that similarities in sequence between foreign (for example, microbe-derived) and self antigens leads to cross-reactive immune responses. Thus infection with such a microbe may fortuitously activate B or T lymphocytes that also recognize self antigens, leading to an immune attack on the body's own tissues.

Natural killer cell: A type of blood lymphocyte mediating rapid immune responses against virus infections, typically before the T lymphocyte response develops. Unlike T lymphocytes, natural killer cells are not specific for a particular virus but recognize generic changes on the surface of virus-infected cells.

Oncogenes: Normal cell genes that drive cell growth and division. Their expression and actions are counterbalanced by tumour suppressor genes whose purpose is to inhibit cell proliferation. An imbalance between these opposing two sets of genes may result in uncontrolled cell proliferation leading to cancer.

Progenitor cell: The stage of development between a stem cell and a fully differentiated cell with the capacity to expand into a clone of identical cells. In the context of cancer, the term typically refers to the identity of the cell from which a monoclonal tumour develops.

T cell/lymphocyte: A type of lymphocyte that generates the specific cell-mediated immune response to, for example, a virus infection. Subsets include (1) 'helper' T cells that help both antibody and 'killer' T cell responses to the infection, and (2) 'killer' (cytotoxic) T cells that kill virus-infected cells.

Viral capsid antigen: A complex of EBV-encoded proteins, all made during virus replication, which assemble to form the virus capsid. (See Capsid)

Viral Envelope: A membrane that, in certain virus families including the herpesviruses, forms the outer face of the virus particle.

X chromosome: The female sex-determining chromosome. Females have inherited two copies of the X-chromosome, one from each parent; males have inherited one X chromosome from their mother and a Y-chromosome from their father.

TIME LINE OF KEY DISCOVERIES RELATING TO EPSTEIN-BARR VIRUS

1958—Denis Burkitt described a tumour in African children now known as Burkitt Lymphoma. He went on to show that the tumour incidence was geographically restricted to regions with high temperature and rainfall. This suggested that, like malaria and yellow fever, the tumour was caused by an infectious agent with an insect vector. (*Chapter 1*)

1964—Anthony Epstein and Yvonne Barr found a 'new' virus in Burkitt lymphoma cells now known as Epstein-Barr virus or EBV. Subsequent work showed that almost all cases of African Burkitt lymphoma contain the virus genome. (*Chapters 2 and 4*)

1966—First evidence of a link between EBV and nasopharyngeal carcinoma (NPC), a tumour located at the back of the nose and very common in southern China. It is now known that every cell in 100% of NPC tumours worldwide contain the virus genome. (*Chapter 5*)

1968—EBV infection shown to cause infectious mononucleosis (glandular fever), a common illness in adolescents and young adults. The virus is spread in saliva and so the disease is commonly known as 'the kissing disease'. (*Chapter 3*)

1975—EBV infection shown to cause a rare, inherited, fatal form of infectious mononucleosis in boys, now called x-linked lymphoproliferative syndrome. (*Chapter 6*)

1978—Large field studies in Africa showed that children developing Burkitt lymphoma could be distinguished from control children by very high levels of antibodies to EBV present for several years before the tumour appeared. (*Chapter 4*)

1980—EBV found to cause lymphoma in recipients of organ transplants who are immune suppressed to prevent organ rejection. (*Chapter 6*)

1984—The complete EBV genome sequenced. This led to identification of EBV 'oncogenes' - virus genes that drive cells to grow and, on rare occasions, to cause cancer. (*Chapters 6 and 9*)

1987—EBV found in Hodgkin Lymphoma. It is now known that around 50% of Hodgkin Lymphoma cases globally are associated with EBV. (*Chapter 7*)

1988–1990—EBV found in rare tumours of T lymphocytes and of natural killer cells, most often seen in South-East Asian people. (*Chapter 7*)

1995—First successful use of immune T lymphocytes to treat an EBV-associated cancer, the lymphoma appearing in immune-suppressed transplant recipients. (*Chapter 8*)

2007—First control trials of an EBV vaccine in humans. This research is still ongoing using new animal models to determine the optimal strategy for prevention of EBV-related diseases. (*Chapter 8*)

2000–2010—Mounting evidence of a link between EBV infection and multiple sclerosis. (*Chapter 9*)

INDEX